PRAISE FOR
SECRETS OF SELF-HYPNOSIS

"Very inspirational and thought-provoking. It offers an opportunity to improve your intellectual and creative potential and, thus, help you achieve and experience much more success and happiness in life than you ever dreamed possible."

—Dr. Frazier Douglass,
Professor of Psychology, Athens State University

PRAISE FOR
PSYCHIC EMPOWERMENT FOR EVERYONE
by Joe Slate, Ph.D., and Carl Llewellyn Weschcke

"This primer says it all: from metaphysical theory to the science behind it, from personal development to practical application, from accessing our dreams to addressing the challenges of our time with exercises for visioning a positive future. Weschcke and Slate have left a legacy of esoteric knowledge that should become part of everyone's inner development."

—Anodea Judith, Ph.D., author of
Wheels of Life and *Waking the Global Heart*

"From the internationally renowned author of eleven other books on psychic phenomena comes this exciting joint venture—*Psychic Empowerment for Everyone*. This astounding collaboration between Dr. Joe Slate and the CEO of Llewellyn Publications, Carl L. Weschcke, can teach you how to make practical use of the amazing powers that all of us possess. I hope you will give this book the opportunity to transform your life."

—Dr. Penne J. Laubenthal,
Professor Emeritus, Athens State University

"*Psychic Empowerment for Everyone* shows beginning and advanced psychics alike, through unique, practical, and easy mind-opening exercises, how to open the sixth sense and use it to enhance the five senses. Meticulous research by Joe Slate, Ph.D., and straightforward explanations by coauthor Carl Llewellyn Weschcke not only teach readers how self-empowerment is vital to our health and spiritual development, but how it can change the world in which we live."

—Debra Glass, MAed., author of *Mediumship To Go*

"This book is a treasure—everything psychic you want to know or explore is here, in clear language and with plenty of advice and guidance for practicing and obtaining results. Buy this book and practice, practice, practice."

—José Feola, Ph.D., author of *PK: Mind Over Matter*

"Thought has power—Weschcke and Slate show this vividly in *Psychic Empowerment for Everyone*. Here is the common sense of psychic power: self-hypnosis and control of the imagination focus plans for success. All of us need it."

—Noel Tyl, author of *Solar Arcs* and
Noel Tyl's Guide to Astrological Consultation

SECRETS OF
SELF HYPNOSIS

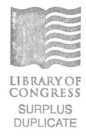

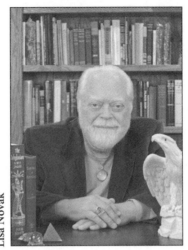

Lisa Novak

Carl L. Weschcke was the Chairman of Llewellyn Worldwide, Ltd., one of the oldest and largest publishers of New Age and occult books in the world. Weschcke (a Magician, Student of Tantric Philosophy and of Western Magic, and former Wiccan High Priest) played a leading role in the rise of Wicca and Neo-Paganism during the 1960s and 1970s, purchasing Llewellyn Publications in 1960.

A life-long student of a broad range of New Age and Occult subjects, Weschcke studied with the Rosicrucian Order, the Society of the Inner Light, and explored studies and practical research in Tantra, Taoism, Kabbalah, Astrology, Shamanism, Wicca, Magic, Psychology, and Spirituality.

In addition to an academic degree in business administration, he held a certificate in clinical hypnosis, and honorary recognitions in divinity and magical philosophy.

In addition, he devoted time to studying quantum theory, Kabbalah, self-hypnosis, and psychology, and to writing. He passed from this realm in 2015.

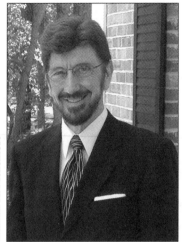

Joe H. Slate, Ph.D., is a licensed psychologist and Emeritus Professor of Psychology at Athens State University in Alabama. The U.S. Army and the Parapsychology Foundation of New York have funded his lab projects in parapsychology. His research led to the establishment of the International Parapsychology Research Foundation. Dr. Slate has appeared on several radio and television shows, including *Strange Universe* and *Sightings*.

SECRETS OF SELF HYPNOSIS

harnessing the enormous
potential of the mind

CARL LLEWELLYN WESCHCKE
JOE H. SLATE, PH.D.

Llewellyn Publications
Woodbury, Minnesota

First Edition
Second Printing, 2019

Orginally published in 2010 as *Self-Empowerment through Self-Hypnosis*

Cover design by Shira Atakpu
Editing by Connie Hill
Illustrations on page 121 and 192 by the Llewellyn Art Department

Llewellyn is a registered trademark of Llewellyn Worldwide, Ltd.

Library of Congress Cataloging-in-Publication Data

Weschcke, Carl Llewellyn, 1930–2015
  Secrets of self hypnosis : harnessing the enormous
potential of the mind / Carl Llewellyn Weschcke, Joe H. Slate. — 1st ed.
      p.   cm.
  Includes bibliographical references and index.
  ISBN 978-0-7387-5941-8
  1. Autogenic training. I. Slate, Joe H. II. Title.
  RC499.A8W47   2010
  615.8'5122—dc22   2009048406

Llewellyn Publications
A Division of Llewellyn Worldwide Ltd.
2143 Wooddale Drive
Woodbury, MN 55125-2989
www.llewellyn.com

Printed in the United States of America

Other Books by Joe H. Slate, Ph.D.

Aura Energy for Health, Healing & Balance
Beyond Reincarnation
Psychic Vampires
Rejuvenation
Connecting to the Power of Nature
The Power of Dreams

Also by Carl L. Weschcke and Joe H. Slate, Ph.D.

Psychic Empowerment for Everyone
Astral Projection for Psychic Empowerment
Astral Projection for Psychic Empowerment CD Companion
Clairvoyance for Psychic Empowerment
Communicating with Spirit
Doors to Past Lives & Future Lives
The Llewellyn Complete Book of Psychic Empowerment
The New Science of the Paranormal
Self Empowerment and Your Subconscious Mind

Also by Carl L. Weschcke and Louis Culling

The Complete Magic Curriculum of the Secret Order G.B.G.

CONTENTS

PREFACE

JUST WHO DO YOU THINK YOU ARE?
THE ANSWER MAY SURPRISE YOU

Who you are—*Who am I?*—is one of the most important questions *you* can ask yourself.

"Know Thyself" (this motto was inscribed on the sixth century BCE temple of Apollo at Delphi) is a familiar bit of advice passed down over the ages because knowing who you are is the first step in self-knowledge and self-understanding, and that itself is the first step in the life-journey of self-improvement that we all *need** to make.

Let's pretend that I'm asking the question. I want to know who the real you is, the self hidden beneath the surface. But the first answer you give to that question is, typically, to tell me things—not about your self, but about your identity. You tell me . . .

Your name, where you live, your age, your educational background, your occupation, your marital status, your children, your parents' national origin, your racial Identity if you wish, your religious affiliation if that's important to you, your political identification if that's important to you, even your social security number. It's like the military response of 'Name, Rank, and Serial Number.'

Yes, you are giving me information about your "identity"—that thing which can be stolen and then give you all sorts of trouble—but you're not telling me anything about the *'self'* you are.

---

* I emphasize need because it is my belief that we are here to grow into 'more than we are,' that it is our life purpose and that which gives meaning to life.

Next, I learn about You, the person, who loves his or her spouse, who is devoted to her or his parents, who avidly watches sports events, who has a small group of very close and supportive friends, who would 'give the shirt off his back' to help his best friend, who has an enduring interest in Celtic spirituality, who reads every news item about paranormal phenomena, etc., but all that is just descriptive and could apply to a whole lot of people. It's just not the 'self' I'm looking for.

I can ask again WHO you are, and I will learn of another person who is of much greater interest to me. This is the person who sets goals for himself and works hard to fulfill them, the person who studies hard and works to improve himself, who is concerned for his personal ability to provide for the health and welfare of his family, and who accepts personal responsibility to help improve the community where he lives. This is the person who sees himself as more than the job he has, as more than the degrees she has earned and the honors she has won, as more than the wealth they may have accumulated, as more than the role she fills, who believes that the world can be a better place and who wants to grow and become more than he is.

Ah. Now I'm beginning to know the real you, that 'self' who is the subject of this book. This isn't your ultimate true self—which we'll reveal later—but it is the self that can be empowered to grow in aptitude, capacity, competence, creativity, and spiritual strength. This is the self that is asking for the power to live this life successfully on its own terms.

It's no small step but a giant leap in personal responsibility and establishment of a life purpose. It is a step toward bringing expanded awareness and higher consciousness into the personality. It's the ultimate meaning of the New Age, that we are evolving into a New Man, a superman in comparison to the ordinary man of a mere hundred years ago.

WHAT IS SELF-EMPOWERMENT, AND WHY IS IT IMPORTANT?

At first glance you may think a definition of Self-Empowerment is easy to give and not of any particular importance to receive. I want to challenge you to change your thinking. Even the definition of "self" is less easy than you may think. "What is 'self'?" And you answer: "That's me. I am my self." As we've just learned, there is more to 'who' you are than 'name, rank, and serial number.' We looked more deeply and arrived at a person interested in personal growth, development, and self-improvement. *Now we have a person who is naturally interested in Self-Empowerment.*

Such empowerment cannot be bought and comes, not as a gift, but through self-discovery and understanding, and then through self-development of the powers innate to the whole person. As you gain knowledge of self, that knowledge—and the power to use it—flows into self. Such power is natural and evolutionary but, historically, it has been suppressed through the denial of knowledge about self and the potentials of the whole person and by the lack of opportunity to move beyond mere subsistence.

No Longer!

In our previous book, *Psychic Empowerment for Everyone,* we revealed the rightful powers and potential of the whole person and how knowledge and understanding will allow those powers to naturally develop and manifest, and we provided exercises for accelerating that development.

In this new book, *Self-Empowerment Through Self-Hypnosis,* we take further steps forward by showing you how to tap into the Subconscious Mind in specific practical applications to recall lost memories and forgotten facts at will, that will enable you to foretell certain coming events, gain information and guidance as needed, develop your innate ESP and PK powers, interact with spirit guides, develop your mediumistic potentials, discover higher planes of power, experience your personal life span—past, present, and future—live younger, longer, and better, accelerate learning and improve memory, manage stress, break unwanted habits, overcome fear, solve problems and resolve conflicts, unleash creativity, manage pain, have a successful career, and achieve mental, physical, and spiritual balance.

You will also learn the principles of hypnotic induction, the key steps (with specific instructions for each) in the induction process, the *I AM* principle of suggestions, and the use of induction aids such as fascination devices, focusing tools, music or sound backgrounds, and counting and visualizing scenes.

Other applications of self-hypnosis/self-empowerment include health diagnosis, healing practices, self-programming for success, building self-confidence, attracting wealth, changing your appearance, building a group mind for team projects, visualizing steps toward a goal, guided meditation, Kabbalistic path-working, using various shamanic practices, astral projection and astral travel to specific destinations in the astral world, and using astral doorways with the Tarot, Runes, and I Ching Hexagrams to access the Collective Unconscious—*the greatest natural resource any of us has*!

Self-hypnosis provides a new generation of people with the power to facilitate the most exciting moment in human history: the true transition from other-directed Piscean Man to inner-directed Aquarian Man.

I believe we will see 'the end of the world as we know it' and the birth of a 'New World Order.' It will be hard to perceive as it occurs because we will be in the midst of it and personal survival for some may be an issue during ensuing natural and man-made disturbances, but if we can look back twenty years from now it will be very apparent. It will be as much—or more—of an inner transition as an outer one.

This may be the meaning of the Mayan prophecy for 2012: that the world, as we know it—the old world of repression and warfare, of egotism and greed, the rape of natural resources, the theocratic suppression of women and use of children as innocent soldiers, and other ugliness we need not repeat here—will be replaced by a New World Order* and global civilization based on a world economy, a common currency, universal education, universal human law, and free trade.

---

* A 'World Order' is the overall structure of the intergovernmental networks of governance, the integration of national and regional economies, the role of international law, the play of communication, and the interrelationships of the dominant cultures. When the existing order is dysfunctional, threatening to tear apart, a new order must replace the old.

I promised a surprise answer to the question of "Just WHO do you think you are?" The true you is without describable characteristics because this you is *pure consciousness*. That's who, or what, you really are: *pure consciousness* on a journey through life, a tiny bit of the universal consciousness that is the inner Divinity that empowers every one of us. And it is through that self-discovery that we can change the world as we know it.

Carl Llewellyn Weschcke
Newport, Minnesota, USA
December 21, 2008

INTRODUCTION

UNDERSTANDING YOUR CONSCIOUSNESS
By Carl Llewellyn Weschcke

Change is a constant. Every second that ticks away brings change; every step we take brings change; things happen to us and we act upon the world around us, always bringing change. We think we're changeless, except for the inevitable changes of growth and decline we know as aging. We are wrong. Every thought, feeling, movement, breath brings change because we are all interrelated not only with other humans but with all life and all consciousness and even all matter and energy, all light and all spirit throughout the universe.

To understand CHANGE itself, and its importance to a richer and better life—both for you and me and for the world we live in—we have to understand your consciousness, what it really is and how it works.

Why? Because consciousness is the beginning, the starting point of everything that is. In the Christian Bible (John 1:1–4), it says:

In the beginning was the Word, and the Word was
with God, and the Word was God.
The same was in the beginning with God.
All things were made by him; and without him was not
any thing made that was made.
In him was life; and the life was the light of men.

Thus, the "word"—*information* or *instruction*—was the beginning of "all things," of "life," and of "the light of men."

START AT THE BEGINNING

The new science of Quantum Theory tells us that the beginning *is* (not just was, *but still is*) the Universal Field of Possibilities that manifests first as Energy/Matter under the guidance of packets of information/instruction. Thus we can see an analogy with a computer with its operating program and its application programs.

The operating program in your computer is analogous to your consciousness. The characteristics, the aptitudes and capabilities you demonstrate are analogous to the application programs. Together, they are the person you are, what we call your "personality." Behind (or above or in another dimension, or wherever you want to think of it) there is another consciousness, pure and with no need for application programs, that we call your "Soul."

The analogy between your personality and the computer doesn't mean that you're only a robot (although, sometimes we do react without thought in robotic ways); rather it gives us a model for self-understanding and for change through self-empowerment affecting the operating program and self-improvements affecting the application programs. Both can be changed, but change comes to the operating system with greater difficulty. We'll discuss that later.

HOW TO SEE CONSCIOUSNESS

The easiest way to "see" something that is invisible and intangible is to build a model in your imagination. The triune model of consciousness we're using applies only to your personal consciousness, your personality. Let's take a look at a dictionary definition of personality: *the totality of somebody's attitudes, interests, behavioral patterns, emotional responses, social roles, and other individual traits that endure over long periods of time.**

You, the person you are—the personality—is made up of:

a. Your awake consciousness that you think of as "my self."

b. Your subconscious mind that you normally encounter, *unconsciously*, only in your sleep and through dreams.

---

* Encarta online dictionary, copyright © 2008 Microsoft Corporation.

c. Your super consciousness that you almost never encounter except through your subconsciousness. And through both the subconscious mind and the super consciousness you can access the collective unconscious with its totality of human knowledge and experience.

This is very simplistic presentation, but it provides all that we need right now. We could draw a picture showing layers, or a round ball of concentric circles, or a kind of pie-chart, but all of them would be limiting, and there is nothing limiting about consciousness—it is everywhere. And even though we discuss it as if there were three or four separate parts, the reality is that this model is only a convenience to our thinking process. To understand, we analyze and break things down into pieces, and then put them back together again. All these parts function together in wholeness. *It is the whole person that we want to empower to live life fully on his and her own terms.*

THE CONSCIOUS MIND—AWAKE AND AWARE

You are awake and aware and, for all practical purposes, "in charge."

In charge of what? That's the question you have to answer. Unfortunately we think we are just our conscious mind, when in reality there are a lot of *hidden* things going on all the time below our immediate awareness.

The conscious mind manages your daily affairs without interfering with the body's autonomic nervous system that safely runs the body functions. Nevertheless, there is a mind-body connection that is somewhat a two-way street. Sometimes mental and emotional stress adversely affects body functions, and other times the body inappropriately affects mind and emotion.

And, just as the body's organs function automatically on their own, so we too have many conscious operations also largely on 'automatic.' We mostly wake up at the same time, eat the same breakfast day after day, and make a routine trip to the workplace, and so on with little conscious effort. Often we only go on to a fully alert (and fully aware) status to handle the exceptional things—as when we run out of the favorite breakfast cereal or some idiot runs a red light. At work we wake up a bit more and function consciously with greater awareness. Other times, and in the evening, we are often in light trances watching sports and game shows on television, carrying on repetitive and bland conversations with family and friends, and sometimes going on full alert to talk politics and money matters with friends and advisors.

Generally, being awake is the same as being aware, but full awareness is more than just being awake, and awareness sometimes occurs even during sleep. Some people have trained themselves to function with awareness while the physical body is asleep. Their awareness works at a low level to perceive minor changes in the environment, and to remember dreams, and can work at a higher level on the astral plane and during out-of-body experiences. Awareness is like a spotlight in the field that is your consciousness: it can light up the whole field, but generally it provides only a gentle background light and an occasional spotlight on areas of interest. Awareness is alertness, concentration, attention, sensitivity, and focus. It is your directed consciousness under control.

Meditation is another time we have a goal of controlled awareness with the physical body at rest. And during hypnosis, awareness is focused on particular goals, sometimes with the body in a sleep state and other times controlling the body in certain physical behavior.

THE SUBCONSCIOUS MIND—
NEVER ASLEEP, ALWAYS AWARE

It's difficult to understand all the ways in which the conscious mind operates and even more so in the case of the subconscious mind. Some people draw pictures of icebergs to point out that the ice beneath the surface is larger than the visible amount above as an analogy with the subconscious below the surface and the conscious above. In other words, we believe the territory we call subconsciousness to be much larger than that of consciousness.

And we say that all the memories you've forgotten are retained in the subconscious and that apparently also includes memories of overlooked details of conscious memories, memories of previous lives and in-between lives.* These memories are much more extensive than those of our conscious mind, filled not only with amazing detail but accompanied by all the associated emotions.

It is helpful to remember that our consciousness arises out of the Field of Universal Consciousness to which we remain connected, and through that we have some degree of connection with all other units of consciousness. Thus the subconscious is also able to access the collective unconscious and at least some elements of the Super consciousness.

ANOTHER PICTURE OF YOUR CONSCIOUSNESS

You may gain a better understanding of your consciousness by picturing it as a large New York City apartment building connected to the life of 'the City' via underground subways, underground communication cables, along with underground pipes and service tunnels supplying fuel, power, and workers to your building. And then, on the first floor of your apartment building, we have a busy lobby with access to street traffic in the front and back, and to other buildings on each side. There are elevators to an underground garage and subways connecting to the rest of the city, and to upper levels where there are skyways connected to other buildings along which there are numerous vendors and public service providers. And up on the roof there are satellite dishes receiving television programming and other wireless communications.

Imagine that on one of the upper floors you have a very large apartment with so many rooms that you've even forgotten some of them that you occupied as a child, others that were once occupied by your parents and grandparents, along with various storage rooms. Even though on the outside this is a very modern-looking building, many of the rooms are far

---

* Newton: *Journey of Souls, Lives Between Lives,* and *Destiny of Souls.*

older than the building. All the rooms at one time were labeled: nursery, Mom's room, Dad's room, Grandpa's room, baby picture storage room, children's toys storage room, Grandma's old clothes store room, and so on. Now, many of the labels have fallen off, and you have no idea what's inside those rooms. Outside of your apartment are corridors leading to your friends' apartments, to the schools you've attended, to several specialized and general libraries, and to offices of your current and past employers along with a police substation, a medical clinic, a psychologist's office, and so forth. In other words, we represent your entire life with this very large building. And, of course, you are fully interconnected with the outside world by your computer and the Internet, and your land and cell phones.

Now, just as many of the city residents believe, we will pretend that New York is the entire world. In its museums you contact all the history, all the culture, all the arts and many ancient artifacts of the world; you have access to theatre, music, operas, schools and universities, experts and special interest organizations of all kinds, the planetarium, the Stock Exchange, the central banking system, many corporate headquarters, botanical gardens, etc. You can visit the United Nations and humanitarian agencies, foundations, and many other important organizations; and you can also find entertainment of all kinds, singles bars, strip joints, underground sex clubs, discussion groups, and more.

In this world of New York, everything imaginable is available, although much is hidden and often overlooked and forgotten about.

With this analogy, we have a picture of your mind—conscious, subconscious, super conscious, the collective unconscious, the connections to other consciousnesses, access to everything you've ever desired or fantasized, and connections to all knowledge, to every kind of expertise, to real benefactors, and to every kind of phony and weirdo.

There is no real limit to the potentials of the human mind but memories do fade, you lose your sense of direction, and the map you once made to some of your apartment's rooms is lost. Sometimes you do wander into an old room with many fascinating memories; other times you find only the most bizarre old clothing, pictures, and letters that you promptly forget about. Sometimes you would like to clean out the old stuff, but then you forget about your plans. Some of the rooms have modern light fixtures, others have none and you need a flashlight if you are searching for something. Sometimes the rooms seem to move about—those you've recently visited move up toward the front and those that are neglected move farther to the back.

You may make an interesting observation: often, when you remember one thing from an old room, memories of other things stored in that same room surface as well. In fact, some of the medieval secret societies taught a technique for memory filing called a "memory palace" in which you learned to visualize rooms in a carefully designed pattern and you would associate learned facts and lessons with similar facts and lessons in assigned rooms. Thus, for example, lessons about alchemy could all be found in the alchemy room, about history in the history room, etc. Each stored memory was thus connected to similar memories and every contact you had with that room strengthened the connections to all the memories.

In a similar vein, many people studying the Kabbalah see the *Tree of Life* glyph with its ten spheres and twenty-two connecting paths as a 'filing cabinet' for you to file corresponding facts and experiences with others of the same nature along with the information similarly filed by millions of other students over hundreds of years.

Everything of your life is here in your building, but you've forgotten what and where many things are. With due diligence, you could map the contents, but you don't really have the time to do it. You'd rather just stay in the few front rooms where you work and play, where you sleep and eat your meals, and where you sometimes entertain guests.

The front rooms represent your conscious mind, and those mostly forgotten back rooms—including the back door leading to the older part of the building—represent your subconscious mind.

ADDING TO THE STORY

Let's continue with our story. Perhaps you form a new relationship that motivates you to find some things from the past and further stimulates you into starting some self-improvement programs. You join one of the nearby gyms and whip your body into shape, and that leads to some new clothes and some other changes in your appearance. You decide to learn the Spanish language and to study Mexican and Mayan history. You and your new friend also plan a vacation to the Yucatan Peninsula and you decide you want to increase your income to better afford your new life style. You take some refresher courses to enhance your professional profile and you join a professional club to increase your business contacts. Then you and your new partner decide to study Mayan shamanic practices together and in the process you meet up with another couple who interest you in Tantra and some Tantric workshops.

All of this new activity gives you a new outlook on life, changing some long-ingrained attitudes and feelings that filter your general perceptions of life and make up your "operating system." And these many self-improvement classes give you new aptitudes that augment your "Application Programs." Along with your new appearance, you gain in self-confidence and have new energy resources. You have more interest in the community and register to vote. You listen to what the candidates say and what the commentators say, and analyze their programs in relation to your needs and ideals. You listen to what your partner says and you both come to some new conclusions.

You have gained in awareness and in doing so you have remembered things from your childhood, things you learned from your grandfather and you remember some experiences with your grandmother who was clairvoyant and a practicing Spiritualist. You are a changed person through your growing self-empowerment.

But there is a big difference between the little bit of unplanned self-empowerment associated with your self-improvement programs and what you can do with the catalytic power of self-hypnosis and direct self-programming that you will learn in this book. We'll explain more about that later, after we complete our introduction of just what consciousness is.

In our discussion of the subconscious Mind with the analogy of the Apartment Building, we have basically pointed to 'lost' or buried memories that can be recalled in meditation and under hypnosis (and in self-hypnosis), but we must also mention its strange ability to override perceptions and sensations of the conscious mind and to sometimes exhibit extraordinary skills and paranormal abilities when in deep hypnotic trance. This is just a hint of the amazing powers of the mind.

FROM CHILDHOOD TO MATURITY

Some of the lost or suppressed memories make up the Shadow. Under hypnosis and self-hypnosis, and in deep meditation and through active imagination guidance, the subconscious is able to telepathically access other subconscious minds and, to some extent, the collective unconscious where we may perceive the Archetypes and gain understanding of our particular interaction with them, and possibly change those interactions from a childish to a more mature level.

In addition to the Shadow, the subconscious contains the Anima or Animus, which is an aspect of self representing the opposite sex, an image often influencing the conscious experience and relationship with a person of the opposite sex, and even more often, unconscious reactions and sexual drives.

PROBLEM SOLVING

The subconscious can solve problems and carry on research projects as directed in meditation or under self-hypnosis. The subconscious mind is also the source of various entities contacted in channeling.

The conscious mind and the subconscious mind, together, are the lower self while the super conscious mind is the higher self. Our goal is to link the two together in wholeness. *It is generally through the subconscious that we access the super conscious mind.*

To finish our analogy between your consciousness and your New York apartment building, let's consider a satellite overhead connecting from the super conscious mind to the subconscious Mind and through to your conscious mind.

THE COLLECTIVE UNCONSCIOUS
Our Inheritance

The collective unconscious is a kind of group mind that is inherited from all our ancestors and includes all the memories and knowledge acquired by humans. It sometimes is called 'the Akashic Records.' These are the enduring records of everything that has ever happened to you, and the repository of all knowledge and wisdom, along with the files of your every personal memory. It is believed to exist on the higher astral and lower mental planes and to be accessible by the super consciousness through the subconscious mind in deep trance states induced through hypnosis, self-hypnosis, meditation, and guided meditation.

Nevertheless, the contents of the collective unconscious seem to progress from individual memories to universal memories as the person grows in his or her spiritual development and integration of the whole being. There is some suggestion that this progression also moves from individual memories through various groups or small collectives—family, tribe, race, and nation—so the character of each level is reflected in consciousness until the individual progresses to join in group consciousness with all humanity. This would seem to account for some of the variations of the universal archetypes each person encounters in life.

The collective unconscious is not something separate from the subconscious mind, nor is its access limited to special people. While it is sometimes imaged as a great library or hall of records, this is a convenience to our consciousness that uses images and symbols much as the computer uses 'icons' to open particular applications.

The Power of Symbols, Images, and Icons

It is through symbols and images, and icons, that we open the doors of our inner perception. The great secrets of magicians, shamans, and modern scientists are in the associations they attach to such icons, and in the power of certain signs and formulae to function as circuits and pathways—not in the brain but in consciousness.

There may be particular 'maps' of these pathways connecting to the powerful symbols and icons that represent particular spiritual traditions and account for their differences in perspectives. And yet the collective unconscious is universal and available to every one of us. Seeing these differences expands our consciousness and broadens our awareness.

THE SUPER CONSCIOUS MIND

The Touch of Divinity

Your subconscious mind is mostly conditioned by the past, and your conscious mind by the present. But you were born with a basic purpose, with some specific learning goals for this lifetime. The Super Conscious Mind is your doorway to and from the future.

But, Past, Present, and Future are not the sum total of your consciousness potential! The super conscious mind is the higher self and the source of your inspiration, ideals, ethical behavior, and heroic action, and the very essence that is "the Light of Men" as it was in the beginning and as it is now and as it will always be . . .

In the core of our consciousness, we have a spark of Divinity that gives us, in our consciousness, the power to shape the future and even to change the present. We will earn that power through the techniques of self-empowerment and the self-improvement programs presented in this book.

WHAT IS AWARENESS? AND WHAT DOES THE ANSWER MEAN?

When we discussed what consciousness is, it rapidly became apparent that "consciousness just IS"! We can't really define consciousness because we are nothing but consciousness, and consciousness cannot really define itself. "I AM THAT I AM."

While we speak of consciousness, subconsciousness, super consciousness and the collective consciousness as if they were separate things or places, they are not. Giving them names and discussing them 'analytically' is just a convenience to allow us to focus our mind on states of consciousness. The same thing happens when we use analogies, such as your apartment and its many rooms in a New York City apartment building with its connections to the world.

Consciousness is not a 'thing' nor is it a function of a 'thing' called the brain. Consciousness is expressed through the brain, but it exists outside the brain. Killing the brain doesn't kill consciousness, but it limits its expression in the familiar physical world.

Awareness, however, is more affected by the limitations of the physical apparatus and the health of the brain. Awareness is the focus of consciousness onto things, images, ideas, and sensations. We are aware of information delivered via our physical senses and our psychic impressions.

Awareness is more than what we sense. We do have psychic impressions independent of the physical apparatus. And we can focus our awareness on memories dredged up from the subconscious; we can focus on symbols and images and all the ideas, and memories, associated with them. We can turn our awareness to impressions from the astral and mental planes, and open ourselves to receiving information from other sources, from other planets, other dimensions, and from other minds as we develop the further resources of our Whole Being.

Awareness is how we use our consciousness. It is just as infinite as is consciousness, just as infinite as is the universe in all its dimensions and planes—and just as *finite* as our self-limiting awareness. When we speak of expanding or broadening our awareness, we are talking about paying attention to new impressions from new sources, and from other ways we can use our consciousness. Awareness is like the operating system we talked about earlier, in that it filters incoming information, sometimes blocking "what we don't believe in."

CHANGE OUR BELIEFS

In other words, to see new things, we often have to change our beliefs—and that can be very, very hard because we sometimes don't really know what we believe.

If we ask you if you believe in "Life After Death," most times you will answer, "Yes, I do." If we then ask, "Do you believe in after-death communication?" you might answer, "My Religion forbids it," or "I'd be too scared," or "No, I don't believe it's possible," or "Not until after Judgment Day." Most of us have been conditioned not to believe in after-death communication and any experience of it is filtered out and denied or associated with negative impressions.

There is another strange thing about belief. Sometimes a whole lot of people have to change their beliefs before new perceptions can happen. Some of it starts in childhood as we listen to our authority figures tell us certain things are impossible, wrong, or forbidden. It can also be that belief is transferred into childhood fantasy—like Santa Claus and his reindeer. As a small child you are allowed to believe in Santa, but children notice that adults smile and have a twinkle in their eye when Santa is discussed, and they rapidly realize that Santa and Cinderella and even Mickey Mouse have a different 'reality' than Mom and Dad. As fantasy, we accept that change in our perception as we "grow up."

Yet, watch a child at play when 'pretend' takes on its own reality. The young lady assembles her dolls for a tea party, and they drink their imaginary tea and converse about important things. For the moment that tea party is just as real as will be the family dinner that evening.

In essence, we change our beliefs only when something new is proven to us and it is accepted by more of the authority figures. And it is "how" we believe that affects what we see. You may believe in life after death and in the possibilities of communication with those who have crossed over, but you might still fear 'ghosts' and hauntings. Your fear will affect what you perceive. Or you may have a very positive belief that when we die in this physical plane, we take on a new life in the spiritual world and are too busy to be dragged back into communication with people in this world.

What and how you believe affects, limits, distorts, or obstructs what you perceive and how you perceive. We need to work directly with the filter, the operating system, to change what and how you perceive, and that you will learn is accomplished with self-empowering self-hypnosis.

WHAT IS TRANCE?

What do you think trance is? You've seen hypnotists put people into trance in the movies, on TV, and maybe on stage. What you've seen has varied from the entranced person being helpless to fend off the advances of Bela Lugosi playing the role of the vampire Dracula, to a young person on stage barking like a dog, and to a person in a hypnotic trance being able to recall forgotten details of a past event. You may have been in a therapeutic situation where you were able to break the smoking habit or to overcome childish fears.

You may think that trance means that you have lost control of your mind and body to another person. You may have seen a film of Voodoo or another religious ceremony in which a person is seemingly possessed by a god, a spirit, or the Holy Spirit. Sometimes a possessed person is capable of feats of the body beyond the normal—as in consuming large amounts of alcohol without effect, walking on hot coals, amazing gymnastics, talking in tongues or another language, having strange fits, and being healed of crippling illness.

A dear friend of mine, Dr. Jonn Mumford, who is also known as Swami Anandakapila Saraswati, is able himself to do remarkable things and to enable others to have amazing experiences with long needles inserted through cheeks and arms, and even tongues without pain, and licking white-hot steel rods without burns. As I watched these things I said to him, "You really are in a trance in which you have moved your consciousness away from the particular physical event so that the body doesn't react." He said I was correct. By directing awareness away from the act, consciousness followed, and without consciousness, nothing could happen.

Trance Is a Focus of Awareness

Now I ask you to listen to your head. *How many conversations are going on in your mind right now? Why aren't you paying attention only to what I'm asking? Here you are reading this book, but how many places have you been mentally in just the last five minutes? Why aren't you here and now, front and center, paying attention to me and no one else?* **You are occupied with 'monkey chatter,' even while reading this excellent book!**

Trance is the focus of consciousness through directed awareness on a single object, person, or idea—or on nothing at all. Trance is not so mysterious, but what is mysterious is that our normal consciousness is so busy with unimportant things. We talk to ourselves, we listen to what others say, we remember conversations from yesterday, we wonder what to have for dinner tonight, we scratch our scalp, we wonder how the stock market is doing, and maybe a dozen other things. With such divisive thinking, is it any wonder that we are not performing miracles!

You don't have to have a crowd of people and uninvited ideas living in your head. Push them away and keep the slate clean except when you invite new ideas in your brain-storming sessions, or as you explore old memories for the single one you are looking for. *Don't waste your consciousness on the uninvited!*

AWAKE OR SLEEPING TRANCES

You can have both a waking trance and a sleeping trance. Whenever you pay close attention to an idea, to conversation, to an object and to your imagination, you are in an awake trance. The greater your depth of attention, the focus of your awareness, the deeper is your trance. The deeper is your trance, the more you are directing your consciousness to the object of your attention. The more directed your consciousness, the more energy is focused on the thought.

A sleeping trance is simply a trance state in which you have given over conscious control to another person, a god, spirit, guide, or 'control'—or a fragment of your own consciousness. You can put yourself into a sleeping trance as we will teach later under self-empowerment through self-hypnosis.

A somewhat different situation arises when the control is involuntary. It becomes a state of possession in which a spirit or other entity, such as a "Loa" in the Voodoo religion, seems to push your conscious to one side and their consciousness takes over your body and personality.

THE INFINITE POWER OF THE IMAGINATION
Your Doorway to the Fulfillment of All Your Dreams

Too often the central role of imagination is downplayed. "It's only your imagination" says you should turn away from using the imagination productively and creatively, leaving it for fantasy only.

Everything starts in the imagination! We don't credit its primary role because we switch terminology and say "we're thinking about it," when what we really are doing is working with the creative power of the imagination to visualize something new. Some definitions of imagination include:

1. **Ability to visualize**: the ability to form images and ideas in the mind, especially of things never seen or experienced directly

2. **Creative part of mind**: the part of the mind where ideas, thoughts, and images are formed

3. **Resourcefulness**: the ability to think of ways of dealing with difficulties or problems

4. **Creative act**: an act of creating a semblance of reality, especially in literature (Encarta Dictionary)

"In the beginning was the Word," and the Word was, and is, information. But information is not just words but the description for a picture, an image that forms around those words, and even an icon that will move a program in your consciousness. The greater the detail in the image, the more real it becomes. And that is the challenge we face.

I've told this tale before, but it remains a wonderful example of the difference between mere words and a detailed image: *Many years ago, an occult author told me that it was his dream to own a Rolls-Royce automobile. That was it; he never said anything about color, or anything about its condition. Years later, not long before he passed away, he called and said he finally had his Rolls-Royce. Upon further discussion I learned that it was old and well used, and didn't run at all. It was actually up on blocks in his back yard. He didn't know if he could afford to repair it, or even yet what repairs were needed. He had gotten what he wished for, but because he only specified the words "Rolls-Royce" he got no more than he'd asked for.*

The imagination is an amazing and powerful part of our consciousness because it empowers our creativity—the actual ability to create. Our educational system does not provide for training the imagination, so it is entirely up to you to learn it yourself. Here are a few simple exercises that will dramatically improve all your skills, and will make your later programs of self-hypnosis powerfully effective.

Training the Imagination

Re-create Your Room. Simply look about the room you are in right now, and any time you have the opportunity in different rooms, then close your eyes and visually recreate it. With your eyes closed and looking at your imagined image of the room, pick out something significant in all six parts of the room: ceiling, floor, and all four walls. Look for colors and shapes, note textures and the play of light and shadow. Estimate the room's measurements and the sizes of objects. Play a game with yourself and pretend you are going to be paid money for everything accurately remembered.

Then open your eyes and look for those significant areas and see how well you did, and even more importantly, how well you did with the areas adjacent to those significant points. Repeat often. Later, when you are away from the room, close your eyes and recreate it again, and when you return, verify as many of the details as possible.

Self-Imaging. Take a simple statement, like "I AM slim," or "I AM strong," and picture yourself accordingly. Do not think of the process of becoming slimmer or stronger, but just a simple image that is you as stated. Now, write a description of what you saw, in detail. Repeat often.

Re-create an Event. Think of a recent event at which you were present, and picture it in detail. See where you were and see what you were doing. See where other people were and what they were doing. Note what people are wearing, and especially jewelry and watches. Now, listen, and hear the sounds and voices of that event.

Re-create a Story. Take a scene from a novel you recently read, and recreate the story in your imagination. Fill in the detail for what wasn't described in the printed version. Add sound effects, listen to the voices, and hear the sounds of the environment. Pretend that you are watching a movie made from the story and see the actors, see their hair, their clothes, how they move, feel their emotions.

Remember the Day Backwards. See yourself as you prepared to go to sleep, undressing from the day, having dinner, coming home from work, finishing up work, your work that day, etc. all the way back to having breakfast, dressing for the day, using the toilet, washing and showering, getting out of bed, and waking up. Note anything you wished you could change, and intentionally do so in your imagination. This especially concerns feelings where you have regret or even guilt for something said or done to others, and hurt and pain from things others said or did to you.

You don't need to carry pain or guilt around with you. Undo these matters in your imagination with strong feelings of intention to remove the pain, whether yours or others. Such emotion is a barrier to your empowerment.

Create a Memory Palace. I mentioned this earlier. Don't use your own living quarters but create an apartment inside a building, and pretend you are both architect and interior designer. Construct and decorate a room for each major category of your life where you will store objects representing actual memories. Have a room representing marriage, for example, and start it with a wedding picture. Add memories using objects even if you have to imagine one, such as a photo you didn't take, and place it appropriately in the room.

Create another room representing your job, another for your hobby, another for each subject you've studied, and so on.

Now, keep adding memories to your palace. As you review your day, select things to be permanently filed for future reference and create an icon to contain everything important about each such thing.

Journal It. These are all exercises that can be continued, but it's these last two that I really recommend becoming a permanent activity. And how will you enable that? *Journal it!* Nearly every self-improvement system, whether it is esoteric or mundane, recommends that you keep a journal or diary. *Why?* Because the act of recording 'solidifies' everything about the recorded event, and what you intend to do about it. If you regret something you said or did, record that you are un-doing it. If you are happy about something and want to affirm it, record that as well. If you met someone of interest you want to know better, record that too.

THE POWER TO CHANGE

The purpose of this book is your self-empowerment. Instead of letting life happen to you, you can make life happen your way. But you have "to take charge," and "state your intentions." Later we will show you more about this, but here is an interesting quotation that shows you how your own thoughts make changes in your brain's circuitry.

Discoveries in neuroscience have revealed a principle called "Wiring is Firing." Basically this means that the more you think a particular thought or have a particular reaction, you are creating a physical pathway in the brain, insuring the continuance of the pattern. By continually thinking a particular thought, you are literally creating the wiring in your brain to sustain this activity. To change the wiring, change the firing. By stopping your thinking about something, you unplug the life force of your attention and the wiring begins to dissolve. Redirect your thoughts towards something healthy, and the wiring will be created to support the activity. It is as if the physical wiring of our brain coalesces around what we think about. Change your thoughts, and your brain makes up changes! (The Pursuit of Happiness" *by David Pond.*)

And, here's another interesting quotation:

The only interesting journey remains the journey deep into the psyche" (Marc Forster, the new director of the next James Bond movie.)

I want to wish you *bon voyage.*

Carl Llewellyn Weschcke

CHAPTER ONE

HISTORICAL AND SCIENTIFIC PERSPECTIVES

Hypnosis is usually defined as an altered state of highly focused attention and increased receptivity to suggestion. From a scientific perspective, it's now generally accepted that appropriately applied hypnosis can facilitate changes in thoughts, emotions, and behaviors as well as in the physical body. Hypnosis is an altered state of consciousness that has demonstrated remarkable effectiveness in controlling habits, reducing anxiety, accelerating learning, recovering lost memories, managing pain, and promoting wellness, to list but a few of its many applications.

Unlike hypnosis requiring the assistance of a trained hypnotist, self-hypnosis is self-induced and self-managed. But when the dots are finally connected, it becomes increasingly clear that *all hypnosis is self-hypnosis.* Whether we label it hypnosis or self-hypnosis, attaining that altered state of increased attentiveness and receptivity is possible only with the active participation of the consenting participant. Even the expert professional hypnotist is usually quick to point out that your best hypnotist exists within yourself. Self-hypnosis puts you in direct touch with that inner trance specialist that is you wanting change and empowerment. While the professional hypnotist may facilitate the process, success in reaching the hypnotic state remains a function of the self. Acquiring effective self-induction skills, however, typically requires practice and experience with a variety of approaches, as we will demonstrate and describe in this book for you to apply in your personal self-empowerment program.

In recent years, self-hypnosis has progressively gained recognition as a highly practical and effective approach for accessing the subconscious, activating its dormant potentials, and focusing them on designated goals. The applications of self-hypnosis are, in fact, so extensive that the limits, assuming they exist in the first place, are yet to be defined. You can, in fact, use self-hypnosis to discover—and in some instances, generate—totally new powers within yourself while increasing your effectiveness in using them to empower your life (Slate 2001). Self-hypnosis is one of the most powerful options known for accelerating your personal growth and actualizing your highest potentials.

HISTORICAL MILESTONES

Since there exists no clear line of demarcation between hypnosis and self-hypnosis, the historical milestones related to hypnosis are just as applicable to self-hypnosis. Spanning centuries, these milestones, when taken together, reflect the enduring relevance of hypnosis. Among the earliest examples are the well-known sleep or dream temples in ancient India, Egypt, and Greece. While commonly called 'sleep' or 'dream temples,' they were actually *trance* temples in which the subject experienced a sleep-like altered state of consciousness in the presence of skilled practitioners. Through the sleep and dream experience, the subject often underwent a transformation and renewal of mind, body, and spirit. Claims of miraculous interactions with higher beings and cures for conditions ranging from blindness to paralysis were not uncommon.

A much more recent landmark with important implications for modern self-hypnosis was the work of the Austrian physician Franz Anton Mesmer (1734–1815). Mesmer developed a theory he called 'animal magnetism,' using actual iron magnets as healing tools to influence what he believed to be a magnetic field surrounding the physical body. The practice, which became known as mesmerism, included passing a magnet (or at times a twig of wood) over a wound to stop bleeding resulting from bloodletting. An investigation conducted by a French Board of Inquiry, which included the American Benjamin

Franklin, concluded that the purported effects of magnets were instead the consequences of the subject's imagination. Franklin's research team concluded that *the healings were due to the patient's own powers,* not those of the magnet. That finding was to become a major step toward the recognition of hypnosis as a scientific approach with potential for self-development and desired change (Ellenberger 1980).

Another major advancement toward the scientific recognition of hypnosis was the work of James Braid, a neurosurgeon popularly known as the 'Father of Modern Hypnotism.' In 1842, Braid attributed the trance state, which he called 'neuro-hypnosis,' to the fatigue of certain brain functions. To induce that fatigue and the consequent trance state, he used prolonged eye fixation, typically on a slowly moving bright object or pendulum. Braid's work shifted the perception of hypnosis away from sleep and toward a physiological conceptualization. He attempted to use it for the treatment of various psychological and physiological disorders, often through post-hypnotic suggestion, albeit without great success. Although Braid rejected Mesmer's concepts, other physicians did experience considerable success using mesmerism. Among them were John Elliotson (1791–1868) and James Esdaile (1805–1859), both of whom reportedly performed painless surgery using mesmerism as an anesthetic (Ellenberger 1980).

But it was the work of Jean-Martin Charcot (1825–1893) that led to a more extensive application of hypnosis in the treatment of various psychological disorders. His use of post-hypnotic suggestion provided a new framework for the application of hypnosis in recovering lost memories and making current memories unavailable to conscious awareness. The early use of hypnosis by Pierre Janet and Sigmund Freud, both students of Charcot, further contributed to the growing popularity of hypnosis. Adding to these early accomplishments were the contributions of many others who would together establish the foundation for the modern, self-empowering applications of hypnosis and self-hypnosis alike (Ellenberger 1980).

MODERN EMPOWERMENT PIONEERS

Among the pioneers noted for their empowering use of hypnosis are:

- Ambroise-Auguste Liebeault (1864–1904), founder of the Nancy school, whose work emphasized the importance of suggestion and a positive and more permissive relationship between the hypnotist and the subject.

- Clark Leonard Hull (1884–1953), regarded by some as the Father of Modern Hypnosis, who concluded that hypnosis is distinctively unlike the sleep state, thus prompting greater interest in the therapeutic applications of hypnosis.

- Milton Erickson (1901–1980), whose innovative concepts and techniques became important influences on modern schools of thought regarding hypnosis. Among his significant contributions was a rapidly induced form of hypnosis called Erickson Hypnosis, which is still in use today.

Aside from the above, there are many other contributors we could mention, but these are among the most important in the early recognition of the empowerment possibilities of hypnosis. As the historical and scientific advancements in hypnosis continued, interest in hypnosis slowly expanded to include self-hypnosis and its applications, particularly toward *self-development and personal empowerment*. That trend was due in large part to the recognition that hypnosis, to be effective, depends not only on the skill of the hypnotist, but even more importantly, on the receptivity of the participant. That recognition placed the participant, rather than the hypnotist, at the center of the induction process. The result was a moving away from an authoritative, often dramatic induction approach that *commanded* the participant to respond toward a more permissive, person-centered approach that *permitted* the participant to respond. That change was based on the premise that *hypnotic suggestions become effective only when accepted and integrated by the receptive participant.*

Given these dynamics, it becomes increasingly clear that the key to successful hypnosis is the self. The "you" as used in hypnosis and the "I" as used in self-hypnosis both address the self as the essential master hypnotist. *Equipped with effective self-induction and management skills, you become empowered to experience that essential part of your being known as your subconscious with its wealth of empowering resources.*

SELF-HYPNOSIS IN THE LAB

The study of self-hypnosis and its relevance to self-empowerment was to become the centerpiece of research conducted under the auspices of the International Parapsychology Research Foundation (IPRF) established in 1970 at Athens State University (then College) by co-author Joe H. Slate, then Chairperson of the Psychology Department. The Foundation from its inception recognized the subconscious as a domain of limitless potential and the higher self as its gatekeeper. Among the Foundation's earliest projects were studies funded by the U. S. Army (Slate 1977) and the Parapsychology Foundation of New York (Slate, 1984). These studies developed the technology and laboratory procedures required for monitoring the physiological correlates of various altered states, including self-hypnosis. In subsequent studies, a variety of self-hypnosis programs were developed and evaluated for effectiveness.

MIND OVER BODY/BODY OVER MIND

The Foundation's early recognition of the power of the subconscious led to several landmark studies on self-hypnosis. Included among them were the placebo effects of self-suggestion (Slate 1988). Commonly called "mind over body," the placebo effect holds that mental factors, including expectations and beliefs, can influence physiological factors.

A common example of mind over body is the trance deepening technique called *hand anesthesia* in which feeling is mentally removed from the hand and then restored through suggestion. The Foundation's studies, while confirming that common effect and its usefulness, also identified a reverse effect called "body over mind," or the effect of physiological factors on mental functions. For instance, chronic physical pain can generate a depressed mental state, whereupon the depressed mental state increases or at least sustains the chronic pain. Consequently, the mental and physical reactions work together to generate a vicious cycle in which each contributes to the other.

Self-hypnosis, it was found, can break that disempowering cycle and reverse its negative effects by working in both directions. It can focus directly on building a more positive mental state to reduce pain, and it can focus directly on reducing pain to create a more positive mental state. The result is an empowered interactive state of both mind and body. The program is called, as you might expect, *Mind Over Body/Body Over Mind*. The step-by-step program, which is detailed in a later chapter, specializes in the use of self-hypnosis in managing pain and promoting wellness.

Given the success of its placebo research program, the Foundation initiated a series of studies that further explored the mind-body interaction (Slate 1996). Throughout its research, the Foundation emphasized the importance of certain pre-induction conditions and safeguards. Included were a controlled environment free of distractions and a built-in feature of each self-hypnosis induction program that empowered the participant to remain in full control and to exit hypnosis at will. Here are a few of the programs that demonstrated remarkable effectiveness and remain in wide use today:

Stress Management: Replacing Tension with Relaxation demonstrates the effectiveness of self-hypnosis in not only reducing stress but extinguishing such related symptoms as fatigue, sleep disturbance, and muscle tension. To induce the trance state, the program uses suggestions that replace tension with relaxation, beginning at the forehead and moving slowly downward. Imagery of a serene nature scene followed by reverse counting is then used to deepen the trance state.

Stop Smoking Now uses a single self-hypnosis session called New Beginning to instantly break the smoking habit. To induce the trance state, the fingers of either hand are first held in a tense, spread position and then slowly relaxed while counting backward from ten to one. The following simple suggestion is then presented: "I am now a nonsmoker." Subsequent sessions can be used to reinforce a powerful anticipation of success that makes the prospect of failure inconceivable.

The New You uses self-hypnosis to manage weight while promoting health and fitness. For induction, the program uses eye fixation on a shiny object, such as a thumbtack situated slightly upward to facilitate the upward gaze along with suggestions of relaxation and drowsiness. With the eyes closed, mental images of the "perfect you" are then formed followed by the suggestion: "This is the true me."

Star Gaze is a multi-purposeful self-hypnosis program that uses the night sky and a selected star as a symbol of limitless mental, physical, and spiritual empowerment. As you focus on the star, peripheral vision is gradually increased to take in the full sky as suggestions of entering hypnosis are presented. This program is especially effective for goals related to personal relationships and career success. It's also recommended for financial success and abundance.

The Crown of Power uses imagination and gestures linked to the "majestic crown" as a universal symbol of power. This program embraces a holistic approach that recognizes the mental, physical, and spiritual components of self-empowerment. To induce the trance state, the program uses hand levitation in which the hand, through suggestion, becomes weightless and gently rises to touch the forehead. The hand is then allowed to return to the rest position as suggestions of going deeper into hypnosis are presented.

LIVING YOUNGER, LONGER, AND BETTER

In recent years, rejuvenation with emphasis on living younger, longer, and better, became a major component of the Foundation's research program (Slate 2001). In contrast to conventional assumptions that aging is essentially an uncontrolled physiological process, the Foundation designed several self-hypnosis programs that emphasized not only living younger and longer, but improving the quality of life as well. Each program is based on the premise that *aging is a complex mental, physical, and spiritual interaction that can be directly influenced through self-hypnosis.*

The new public interest in rejuvenation, defined as living *Younger, Longer, and Better*, has been credited to the "Boomer" generation—which is also that generation most identified with New Age thinking. We have suddenly realized that the old stereotypes associated with growing older do not have to mean senility, dementia, crippling arthritis, deafness, etc. With modern surgical replacements for arthritic knees, shoulders, hips, etc. that are, in fact, nearly as good as natural, with eye surgery to instantly restore sight to people with cataracts and hearing devices to bring sound back for the deafened, pacemakers for the heart, new mobility devices, and other interventions saving countless lives, our attention has turned to early intervention and prevention with better nutrition, specific therapies, and improved lifestyle that have changed the meaning of retirement to that of opportunity for changed careers, an explosion of interest in new education and crafts, travel and sports, and much more.

All of this has brought about a change in attitude. People <u>are</u> living longer, living younger, and living better, and—more importantly—now can see that the 'golden years' can indeed be beautiful years in which to live the meaningful lives they always wanted. *Rejuvenation is no longer a myth but a physical, mental, and spiritual reality.*

These 'golden years' are the years when self-empowerment can lead to mentally guided spiritual renewal and the opportunity to extend awareness into our larger consciousness so that life is perceived as continuous, with the ultimate death (unless that too is defeated) of the physical body just a transition into an immense new other-dimensional field for living.

Among the Foundation's most innovative programs related to rejuvenation is *Rejuvenation through Age Regression* based on the concept that simply experiencing your past peak of youthful vigor during self-hypnosis can be spontaneously rejuvenating.

To induce the trance state, the program uses suggestions of becoming increasingly relaxed accompanied by peaceful mental imagery and reverse counting. To generate the regressed state, the program uses suggestions of traveling back in time to a stage of youthful prime. The program found that simply lingering in that regressed state of peak youthfulness tends to be rejuvenating. During the regressed state, experiences that over time literally accelerated aging are often uncovered, and even reversed Among the examples are unresolved conflicts and repressed psychological trauma that can hasten aging and, in some instances, result in mental distress or physical illness. Chronic anxiety and fatigue were found to be especially common among participants with a long history of inferiority feelings that were all too often associated with early parental rejection. Almost invariably, enlightenment resulting from uncovering the sources of conflicts and inferiority feelings was sufficient to resolve them. During self-hypnosis using this program, the subject was often reunited with an early spirit guide who would provide essential support, guidance, and in many instances, long-term companionship.

COSMETIC AND CORRECTIVE REJUVENATION

Another highly innovative self-hypnosis program developed by the Foundation, now a private organization, is called *Cosmetic and Corrective Rejuvenation*. This program is based on the premise that a vast reservoir of dormant but powerful rejuvenating energy exists in the subconscious. Cosmetic and corrective rejuvenation uses self-hypnosis to tap into that reservoir. Cosmetic rejuvenation is designed to erase the physical signs of aging, whereas corrective rejuvenation focuses on the biological organs and systems underlying aging. With repeated practice of this highly popular program, the rejuvenating effects become so rapidly evident that they speak for themselves.

Experiencing your past lives and lives between them was to become a major focus of the Foundation's research program. Its studies of past-life experiences are based on the simple premise that knowledge, including that from within the self, is empowering. To uncover that knowledge, the foundation developed a research-based self-regression program called *Eye Movement/Reverse Counting (EM/RC)* which combines certain side-to-side eye movements and reverse counting to induce hypnosis (Slate 2008). During that self-induced state, the participant enters the so-called "past-life corridor" with doors situated on each side. During that regressed state, the participant selects a door to experience the past life it represents. At the corridor's end is a distant door that represents the participant's life before the first lifetime. The EM/RC program includes all the required safeguards to ensure productive retrieval of past-life experiences from the earliest to the most recent lifetime.

PARANORMAL SKILLS

Other Foundation programs focused on the development of various paranormal skills, including telepathy, clairvoyance, precognition, mediumistic communication, psychokinesis, out-of-body travel, and remote viewing, to list but a few. Each program was designed to fit the underlying dynamics of the phenomenon being studied. In the controlled lab setting, performance on each task noticeably improved following self-hypnosis that appeared to activate the subconscious faculty related to it. A prominent feature of each self-hypnosis program was the use of post-hypnotic cues formulated to later activate a particular psychic function on demand.

Eventually, all roads lead to *spirituality*. The road can become temporarily blocked, it can have many twists and turns, and it can even require an occasional detour. Although the road can become bumpy and uncertain, it points always to spirituality and the actualization of our spiritual potential. Even roads that begin in the laboratory ultimately reach into spirituality. Our studies of reincarnation, the out-of-body experience, and life after death led invariably to the inescapable conclusion that *we are by nature spiritual beings*. A look backward reveals a spiritual past; a look forward reveals a spiritual future; and a look inward reveals a spiritual essence without which we would not exist.

INTERDIMENSIONAL INTERACTION PROGRAM

Nothing more clearly illustrates the spiritual essence of our existence than our capacity to interact with the spirit dimension. Our awareness of spirit guides and, in some instances, the departed, illustrates our capacity as spiritual beings to interact with the spiritual realm and gain insight from it. To explore that interaction and its empowering potentials, the Interdimensional Interaction Program was formed at Athens State University under the auspices of the Foundation. A major objective of the program was to determine the relevance of self-hypnosis to spirituality, to include mediumistic communications.

Early on in our research, it became evident that the *mediumistic potential exists to some extent in all of us* as a part of our makeup as spiritual beings. Furthermore, it became clear that we can activate that potential through self-hypnosis using the simple post-hypnotic suggestion: "Upon exiting the trance state, my mediumistic powers will be at their peaks." Not unlike the results of other programs related to the afterlife, many of the participants of this program discovered during self-hypnosis their personal spirit guides and established a long-term interaction with them. This approach was also effective when used to explore the nature of life after death and the purpose of various unexplained discarnate manifestations. Interestingly, this program revealed *no evidence of malevolent beings or evil forces in the after-life realm.* Fears of dangerous consequences of interacting with the discarnate realm appear to have absolutely no basis when viewed in the light of objective research findings.

We will later explore in depth a wide range of self-hypnosis programs now available to promote your personal development and empower you with success in achieving your highest goals. We will specify the steps required for successful self-hypnosis and develop appropriate suggestions for each application.

SUMMARY AND CONCLUSIONS

We are at a stage in human progress and evolution when self-empowerment is called for to continue the Great Adventure and to fulfill the Great Plan. No longer is our lifespan one of birth, procreation, drudgery, senility, and death. Instead we are born, educated, get married, raise a family, and work at jobs often of our own choice. Even while working we can explore beliefs and ideas new to us. We retire and take on new opportunities to grow and expand our horizons, and all the while we enjoy the adventure of life and love.

Human progress is not merely a technological miracle, but is the human miracle of mind and spirit becoming free of the old hypnosis imposed by the outer reality of the physical environment and social conventions and using the new self-hypnosis to shape our own realities to become more than we are. We are no longer slaves, drudges, victims, and people simply locked into class or caste by an archaic system, but now are masters of our own universes expressing the divinity we were given at the beginning.

Self-Empowerment through Self-Hypnosis is the master key to self-liberation and self-fulfillment that bespeaks the end of the old world and the beginning of the new, unfettered to past history.

Note: Both the American Medical Association (AMA) and the American Psychological Association (APA) have endorsed the use of hypnosis and self-hypnosis while emphasizing the importance of appropriate training and continued research. APA has also published several books on spirituality and its relevance to psychotherapy. Among them is a book by William R. Miller (1999) that re-establishes the importance of integrating spirituality into mainstream psychological practice.

REFERENCES AND SUGGESTED READING

Baker, R. *They Call It Hypnosis.* Buffalo, NY: Prometheus Books, 1990.

Ellenberger, H. *The Discovery of the Unconscious.* New York: Basic Books, 1980.

Erdelys, M. H. *The Recovery of Unconscious Memories.* Chicago: University of Chicago Press, 1996.

Miller, W. *Integrating Spirituality into Treatment.* Washington, DC: American Psychological Association, 1999.

Slate, J. *Beyond Reincarnation: Experience Your Past Life and Life Between Lives.* Woodbury, MN: Llewellyn, 2008.

———. *Investigations into Kirlian Photography.* Athens, AL: Athens State University, 1997.

———. *The Kirlian Connection.* Athens, AL: Athens State University, 1985.

———. *Psychic Empowerment for Health and Fitness.* Woodbury, MN: Llewellyn, 1996.

———. *Psychic Phenomena.* Bessemer, AL: Colonial Press, 1998.

———. *Rejuvenation: Strategies for Living Younger, Longer, and Better.* Woodbury, MN: Llewellyn, 2001.

CHAPTER TWO

SLEEP AND DREAMS

Since we spend on average of about a third of our lifetime in sleep, it should come as no great surprise that healthful sleep is essential, not only to our physical health and survival but our total development as well.

In this chapter we are discussing sleep and the dream state from a number of perspectives, including:

- Sleep as a physical necessity, and how to sleep better.
- Sleep as a doorway to the subconscious, and how to best use this doorway.
- Dreams as windows to the subconscious, and how to look through these windows and understand the scenes.
- Dreams as a method of communication with the subconscious mind, and how to dream true.
- How to turn on dream power to answer questions and provide guidance in your life.
- How to interpret dreams.

THE RECUPERATIVE POWER OF SLEEP

While no one really disputes the physical necessity of sleep, there has long been debate about how much sleep is needed, and how one may learn to sleep more efficiently. It is believed, for example, that George Bernard Shaw and Thomas Edison—both intellectual powerhouses—slept only a few hours nightly, although both took short naps during the day. It has also been established that an hour of mindless meditation can substitute for two or three hours of ordinary sleep.

Healthful renewal through sleep empowers us to cope more effectively with the dizzying speed and uncertainties of modern life. In the career setting, it can equip us to meet the demands of breakneck technological advances for which we may be ill prepared. At yet another level, healthful sleep can promote resolution and renewal when hardships occur or trustful relationships rupture. The revitalizing effects of healthful sleep can help ease the feelings of failure all too often associated with career setbacks and ended relationships. We become empowered through healthful sleep not simply to muddle through difficult situations, but to set our sights on the best that can happen rather than the worst. We see a clearer picture, one depicting success rather than failure in a world filled with both challenges and possibilities.

Our attitude toward sleep can affect how we sleep. Many people simply drift off to sleep while reading, watching television, or 'daydreaming.' Other people approach sleep with the intention of 'getting over it' as fast as possible and programming themselves to fall asleep rapidly. And those short daytime naps are often very efficient in fulfilling the physical needs for recuperation.

THE PSYCHOLOGICAL NECESSITY OF SLEEP

Sleep seems to be as necessary from an emotional perspective as from the physical. Failure to renew ourselves through restful sleep can weaken our capacity to meet even the routine demands of daily life. The disruption of normal sleep can result in anxiety, fatigue, irritability, difficulty concentrating, and depression. The loss of sleep when prolonged can severely disrupt psychological organization and generate such symptoms as depersonalization, disorientation for time, person, and place, and, in some instances, paranoia. Even our sanity, it seems, depends on healthful sleep.

Once again, attitude makes a difference. Perceiving sleep as a necessity and going at it as smartly as planning a nutritionally balanced meal rather than fretting and letting worries and concerns disrupt a good sleep brings emotional benefits right along with the physical. On the other hand, once the physical and emotional requirements for sleep have been met, there seems little to be said for a distinct *mental* requirement. The mind can continue functioning through sleep time, solving problems, awakening our subconscious memories, and accessing the collective unconscious.

As expected, individuals including children differ in the amount of sleep they require, with some requiring long periods of uninterrupted sleep while others prefer only brief periods of sleep interspersed over time. Aside from these time differences, the ranges in brainwave activity can vary widely among individuals, not only for sleep but for other states of consciousness as well. For instance, our biofeedback studies found that the beta state of ordinary alertness and concentrated mental activity typically ranges from 14 to 22 Hz. The alpha or relaxed wakefulness state can range from brainwave levels of 8 to 14 Hz. Our studies found that you can easily induce the alpha state by simply settling back, closing your eyes, and rolling your eyeballs gently upward. The theta state of drowsiness and dreaming can range from levels of 4 to 8 Hz, whereas the deepest stages of sleep can range from 0.5 to 4 Hz. As an interesting footnote, the characteristics of sleep vary not only among human beings but other species as well. While we sleep with the whole brain, certain animals, including the iguana, sleep with half the brain and one eye open for protection purposes.

Still, we have every right to ask, "Isn't there a better use for one-third of our total lifetime than *unconsciousness?* I work 40 hours but I sleep for 56 hours a week; I probably spend 28 hours just getting dressed, going to the bathroom, getting undressed, reading the mail, etc., and 31 hours driving to and from work, having breakfast, lunch and dinner. That's 155 hours out of 168 hours of the week! That leaves just 13 hours—less than two hours a day—for me. Sure, I can multi-task a little—watch the news during breakfast, read a newspaper during lunch, talk with my spouse and family during dinner, perhaps I am one who can read while commuting to work—but not if I'm driving! And, yes, I can read in the bathroom, sing in the shower, play with the cat while dressing, *but can't I do more with my sleep time than just recuperate?* What about my consciousness? Why can't we put the body to sleep and keep the consciousness active? Why can't we separate consciousness from the body? Can't there be more than dreams we usually can't understand?"

THE SLEEP DOORWAY TO THE SUBCONSCIOUS

Yes, we can make our dreams more meaningful, we can ask our subconsciousness to learn things and to find information that we need in our awake time, and we can send our consciousness to explore other realities. We can do these things, but we have to understand the possibilities and learn the techniques. Our education is lacking but we can change that: we can extend our awareness into the sub and super areas of consciousness and into the collective unconscious with simple methods we explore in this chapter and again in chapter six.

The difference comes with intent. When we plan our actions with the intention of securing particular benefits, those actions deliver results efficiently and effectively. Sleeping and dreaming are important activities in which we make substantial investments in time (an average of 56 hours weekly) and usually several thousands of dollars in space and furniture.

Understanding their function and planning our sleep and dream work with as much care as we do body work and our professional or educational work will benefit the whole person. Sleep is a doorway into the subconscious mind and dreams are windows into unconscious processing of our requests.

PRE-SLEEP INTERVENTION

Although the stages of sleep are generally seen as essentially different from hypnosis, the drowsy, hypnagogic state between full wakefulness and deeper sleep can be arrested and applied as a trance state with nearly unlimited empowerment possibilities. Programs have, in fact, been developed by the Foundation at Athens State University to do just that. Among the most effective is the "Pre-sleep Intervention Program," which is based on the premise that consciousness and subconsciousness, rather than simply categories or content areas, are complex mental processes that exist on a continuum that is receptive to our intervention.

Through pre-sleep intervention, you can tap into that continuum in ways that influence those processes. As a result, you access dormant potentials and activate them to achieve your personal goals. Beyond that, you can actually generate totally new potentials by taking command of the resources within. By perceiving consciousness and subconsciousness as a continuum, we are activating the 'Whole Person' rather than seeing division and separation. In the following program, the most important step is before the beginning—that you really know what your goal is, or what your goals are. Only work with one at a time but know that it is a vitally important goal and truly <u>feel</u> its importance and value. Be willing to say to yourself that you are wholeheartedly *praying* for its realization. Here's the program:

Step 1. Before falling asleep, formulate a personal goal, write it down, and state your intent to use the drowsy, hypnotic-like state preceding sleep as a gateway to the resources required to achieve it. You know that sleep is a gateway to the subconscious, and that the subconscious has the power and resources to bring your goal into realization. Continue to reflect on your goal, using visualization if possible, as drowsiness slowly ensues.

Step 2. As you become increasingly drowsy, re-state your goal in positive, personal terms and affirm your intent to achieve it. As before, use visualization if possible to give mental substance to your stated goal. For instance, if your goal is rejuvenation, visualize yourself at your peak of youth as you affirm, "*I AM fully infused with youth and vigor.*" Know that your vision is true and that it is the matrix from which reality manifests.

Step 3. As drowsiness further deepens, affirm that as you sleep, your conscious and subconscious powers will interact to fully infuse your life with success, happiness, and abundance. Sense the balance and attunement accompanying the flow of energy deep within as you drift into healthful sleep. As you drift into sleep, sense the emergent sense of oneness, balance, and attunement throughout your total being.

Step 4. Upon awakening, again restate your goal and affirm, "I am empowered with complete success."

With practice using this program, you will become increasingly effective in accessing the subconscious resources related to your stated goal. Should you find the drowsy state too fleeting, you can delay sleep by using the so-called *finger spread gesture* in which the fingers of either hand are held in a spread position throughout the procedure. Another option is the *arm lift*, in which either arm is held in a slightly raised position. Upon relaxing the hand or arm, the drowsy state will typically give way to restful sleep.

Alternatively, knowing that the sleep state unifies the consciousness continuum, you can <u>will</u> yourself to quickly fall asleep as you rapidly move through steps one through three. Recognize this as an active program of moving through changing states of consciousness to accomplish your goal.

YOUR SUBCONSCIOUS RESOURCES

Because is designed to access a vast reservoir of subconscious resources, it is applicable to a near-unlimited range of goals. Rejuvenation, however, is one of its most popular and effective applications. A few moments devoted nightly to this program will generate powerful rejuvenating changes in physical appearance and mental processes alike. The body becomes more youthful in appearance, and such cognitive functions as memory and analytical thinking are markedly improved. In formulating your rejuvenation goals, you can focus on highly specific physical or mental factors, such as the removal of facial age lines or increased ability to recall names. A bridal shop manager insists that she removed the puffiness from under her eyes through repeated use of this program, which included imagery of her face without that feature. Although the puffiness is now gone, she continues to use the program because, in her words, "It's a good way to go to sleep."

And she is correct. Moving rapidly into the sleep state with your goal strongly visualized activates your consciousness continuum in amazing ways. One of your authors lives in a cold climate where winter temperatures well below freezing are common. As a young man, he made control of the body his goal and slept naked beneath only a single sheet in an unheated room with the windows open. It was possible only by instantly falling asleep, and in the morning instantly waking and getting the window closed and the heat on!

Aside from rejuvenation, this program has been highly successful for such diverse goals as losing weight, quitting smoking, increasing creativity, building self-esteem, and improving performance skills. Students have found it remarkably effective in accelerating learning and improving their academic performance in courses ranging from organic chemistry to art appreciation. A psychology graduate student, by her report, used it to acquire in record time a mastery of statistical analysis, one of the requirements for her doctoral degree. She included a suggestion in step three of the procedure that during sleep, her subconscious would work with her in accelerating her mastery of statistics. By her report, she experienced recurring dreams of solving statistical problems with ease and understanding. Her fiancé, likewise a doctoral student, used the program to formulate a highly innovative research proposal for his dissertation. His ensuing research on therapeutic spirituality, according to his doctoral committee chair, "contributed significantly" to the field of knowledge.

Another college student majoring in elementary education used it to secure a third-grade teaching position at the school where she had completed her internship. In step two of the program, she visualized the familiar classroom setting while affirming, "This is my classroom and these are my students." She is today the principal of that school.

A high school coach, who himself had used the program to improve his golf game, oriented his basketball team regarding its effectiveness and suggested they consider using it to improve their performance. He recommended powerful affirmations of success accompanied by visualization of a performance standard he called *Perfection in Playing the Game.* It apparently worked. His team enthusiastically applied the program and became the regional champion.

DREAM INTERVENTION

Dreams are among the most common manifestation of the subconscious, that vast domain of experiences that stretches from your earliest pre-existence to the present. Through your dreams, you can get glimpses of that immense repository that includes your experiences of past lifetimes as well as those critical intervals of experiences between lifetimes. Aside from these, you can recover those unknown present life experiences, including your prenatal existence, birth, and very earliest childhood. Through your dreams, you can even get glimpses into your future, including your life after death.

In addition to its critical function as a valuable reservoir of past experience, the subconscious is a dynamic, interactive process. It interfaces conscious awareness, and constantly interacts with it. It can facilitate problem solving, generate creative ideas, offer spontaneous protection through a variety of defense mechanisms, and strengthen our ability to meet challenges and overcome difficulties. It can psychically access the future and generate awareness of far distant conditions. It can interact with higher dimensions of reality to gain new knowledge and power. It can function as a channel for direct communication with the spirit realm, channeling other intelligences and facilitating spiritual interactions.

The subconscious, like life itself, is a continuous work in progress with resources that are available to you at any moment. It persistently beckons your interaction, albeit indirectly through such experiences as intuitive awareness, flashes of insight, unexplained awareness of future events, and peak moments of enlightenment and power, to list but a few. The Dream Intervention Program is designed to facilitate productive interactions with the subconscious by focusing on the dream experience as a channel. This program is based on the premise that subconscious powers seek our awareness and interaction through our dreams. Through deliberately intervening in the dream experience, we can access relevant knowledge and activate the subconscious powers related to our present life situation and goal strivings.

Let's step back for a moment and consider how we think about our goals. Aside from purely spiritual goals, most fall into three primary categories relating to pleasure, power, and happiness. The first two can be visualized as richly sensual or ego aggrandizing. Pleasure, which encompasses sexuality as well as other aspects of sensuality, is experienced with the body *turned on*—glowing with excitement. Power is experienced with the mind *turned on*—enjoying the respect of others.

Happiness is an all-inclusive category. The statement: "I AM happy" is so positive that it readily brings a smile to your face. It's as if the Spirit is *turned on*.

The Dream Intervention Program recognizes that your most proficient healer, therapist, and teacher exist within yourself, responsive to your desires. They are part of the Whole Person you are. Through this program, you can directly experience them and activate their powers. You can focus their powers on specific goals, whether mental, physical, or spiritual. Here's the program.

Step 1. Relax your body and calm your mind. Put aside all worries, concerns, and even pleasant fantasies. Sleep is a purposeful activity of physical recuperation and mental access to the subconscious world of knowledge and power. Your dreams are dramas in which your goals will be fulfilled. Visualize them accompanied by those body, mind, or spirit associated feelings just mentioned.

Step 2. As you prepare for sleep, take a few moments to recall your personal goals and your intention to use sleep and dreams as sources of power. Let peaceful images, including those related to your goals, spontaneously flow in and out of your mind. Let yourself become increasingly comfortable and relaxed as the images come and go.

Step 3. As drowsiness ensues, let yourself go to that quiet place deep within yourself. Sense the peace and serenity of that innermost space as the center and essential essence of your being. Think of it as your connection to the highest realms of power, a place without limitations. As you linger in that bright space, affirm that as you sleep, your dreams will be a source of enlightenment and power. Tell yourself that whatever you need at the moment is now available to you through your dreams.

Tell yourself that as you sleep, you will be empowered to intervene into the dream experience and focus your dreams on your desired goals. Further affirm that upon awakening, you will recall your dream experiences and understand their relevance.

Step 4. Let dreamlike images and impressions unfold as you drift deeper into sleep. As your dreams unfold, let yourself flow with them while intervening as needed to shape and direct them toward your personal goals.

Step 5. Upon awakening, record your dream experiences in a dream journal and reflect on their significance. Pay particular attention to the feelings associated with body, mind, or spirit.

DREAMS AS WINDOWS TO THE SUBCONSCIOUS

Through this program, you can activate your subconscious powers, to include those directly related to your personal goals. By acknowledging the dream state as part of the continuum of consciousness in which your goals are being manifested, your dreams can become sources of new knowledge and power not otherwise available to you. Among the common examples of spontaneous empowerment through this program is the liberating effect of past-life enlightenment. For instance, a young auto mechanic whose fear of crowds was so intense that he avoided even family gatherings experienced during dreaming a distant past life in which he was clubbed to death by a primitive tribe. With that insight, his fear of crowds eased and soon vanished altogether. A single flash of insight through dreaming was sufficient to liberate a lifetime (or possibly many past lifetimes) of fear.

In another instance of the liberating power of dreams, a student whose fear of flying seriously limited his life decided to use the Dream Intervention Program to focus dreaming on the source of his fear. During dreaming, he experienced a past life that ended when he was pushed from a cliff to his death. His awareness of the past-life source of his fear instantly extinguished the mystery and irrationality of the fear along with the fear itself.

Interactions with higher dimensions of power often accompany this program. A student whose grandmother was on life support in a critical comatose state experienced during sleep the presence of her grandmother in a radiant garment, ascending slowly with what appeared to be two angels, one on each side. The student, by her report, felt herself leaving her own body and slowly ascending to join her grandmother at a distance in the company of the angels. She embraced her grandmother and continued to ascend until one of the angels spoke, "You must now return. It's not yet your time." She then slowly returned to her body at rest. Fully awake, she immediately called the hospital and was informed that her grandmother was still on support but at the edge of death. Within hours, her grandmother died. The student, however, remains convinced that she accompanied her grandmother on her transition to the other side prior to her bodily death.

This student's account begs the twofold question: *Can we experience the after-life realm in the out-of-body or astral projected state, and, equally as important, can our transition to that realm occur before bodily death is complete?* There's a gathering body of evidence suggesting that both are possible, as well as the actual re-engaging of the physical body following the partial- or near-death experience. There is, however, little evidence other than fictional or mythological supporting the possibility of returning to reunite with the physical body after full death. There is, of course, a mountain of evidence supporting the possibility of the departed to re-engage physical reality, often to interact with those left behind. The countless reports of ghosts and hauntings offer additional evidence of the capacity of the departed, including animals, to re-engage this physical reality, always with purpose yet, unfortunately, not always with the full acceptance and understanding of those left behind.

One view of sleep holds that sleep itself is an out-of-body state in which the astral or nonbiological body disengages the physical body and hovers over it during sleep. An extended view of that concept holds that during sleep, the astral body becomes liberated to travel to distant realities, including the spiritual, and interacts with them. That view holds that out-of-body visitations during sleep are, in fact, common and, for the most part, purposeful. For instance, out-of-body visitations to a place of previous employment can ease the anxiety of job change and promote adjustment to a new work situation. Similarly, out-of-body interactions with family or friends at a distance can help satisfy the need to stay in touch beyond simply text messaging and calling by phone.

DREAM COMMUNICATIONS

Based on numerous case reports, out-of-body interactions during sleep can reach far beyond merely observing distant realities. They can include profound interactions that meet both mental and physical needs. A former student and research assistant who is now in the military insists that he visits regularly with his wife at a designated time and place where they interact both mentally and physically. They each use the Dream Intervention Program, which he incidentally helped to develop, to initiate out-of-body travel.

Again, based on numerous case reports, this program is among the best available for initiating productive interactions with the spirit realm. Even in the absence of stated goals, reports of interactions with spiritual planes as well as personal spirit guides are common. In step 4, you can experience awareness of various spiritual planes of color and yourself interacting with them, often bathing in their energies. The color of the various planes offers a clue to their empowering qualities. By interacting with bright planes of green, you can infuse yourself fully with healing and rejuvenating energy. You can interact with planes of gold to accelerate learning and improve the rate of learning, including mastery of new languages, which seems particular receptive to this plane. You can interact with planes of purple for spiritual and philosophical enlightenment. Planes of blue are associated with serenity and well-being. By interacting with the various planes of color through this program, you can become attuned, balanced, and empowered mentally, physically, and spiritually. Nothing is beyond your reach when you are infused with the multiple powers of the spirit realm.

Perhaps not unexpectedly, personal spirit guides can come forth during this program, at times with what seems to be healing energy. An engineer who had participated in our early dream research experienced a direct interaction with a spirit being in step 2 of the procedure as he lingered in the trancelike hypnagogic state. The guide, enveloped in a shimmering green radiance, reached forth and gently touched the engineer's forehead. The engineer, who had been diagnosed with liver cancer and was scheduled to undergo surgery, experienced instant warmth that spread from his forehead downward and throughout his full body. Additional diagnostic tests conducted a few days later showed no signs of cancer. The intervening guide would become, by his report, a lifelong companion who continues to enrich his life.

DREAM POWER

We have established that the subconscious Mind is a powerful resource. Perhaps it is the 'missing ninety percent' of our mental capacity that people often quote, matching—in a sense—the missing ninety percent of the Universe sometimes called 'Dark Matter.'

But the subconscious mind is not really a part of us hidden away and neglected in 'the basement' of our personality. Instead, it is in a continuum of our total consciousness that makes up the totality of the whole person, the *holy person*, we are.

The subconscious is with us fulltime, always awake and ready to respond to our beck and call, ready to answer our questions and respond to our directives. Yes, it has been neglected by our educational system; it has been ignored by Church and treated like a displaced person by Authority. Yet, it is totally faithful when given respect and a magical powerhouse when approached with knowledge.

You can plan to use this powerhouse simply by using your journal to write down questions or directives to be answered through dreams. Ask a specific question, or make a positive I AM statement as you enter sleep, and repeat nightly. Treat the answers you get like three-dimensional holographic images to be explored from all angles because you have to build your lines of communication with the Sub-Conscious.

You are employing dream power. And you are learning that the *intentional* use of consciousness in all its states is what self-empowerment is all about.

INTERPRETING DREAMS

Although the messages of dreams can be direct and free of disguise, many of our dreams challenge us not only to remember them but to unravel their true meanings as well. The conscious or manifest content of the dream can represent a complex body of latent or subconscious content. Ironically, the most powerful messages of our dreams are often the most heavily disguised. There is reason, however, behind that irony. *The subconscious seems to know that the greater our effort in uncovering the dream's true message, the more highly motivated we become in applying it.* Here are three of the most commonly used dream mechanisms:

Symbolism. The uses of an object, sign, or signal to represent an idea or action. The meanings of symbols are inexact, often colored by personal experience, and will vary widely. For example, a moving train can represent a spiritual journey, a need to escape, or, from an analytical perspective, sexual gratification; being borne aloft can symbolize freedom from self-imposed limitations or, from a totally different perspective, out-of-body travel; and a mountain can represent challenge, barrier, or aspiration, to mention but a few of the many possibilities.

Condensation. The compression of many ideas or processes into a single object or word. For instance, a book can represent the accumulated wealth of past experiences, a weapon can represent a war, and a house can represent family history.

Antithesis. The use of an object or action to represent its direct opposite. Examples include the use of death to represent life; failure to represent success; and loss to represent gain.

Unraveling the meaning of your dreams can challenge both reason and imagination. It may require reflecting on your past and present life experiences as well as your goals and aspirations. Word association, in which you state a dream object or action and await impressions to spontaneously emerge, can be highly effective in identifying the dream's hidden meanings. Although discovering the dream's true message can require considerable time and persistence, it is well worth the effort. You will eventually discover that your dreams can be important sources of knowledge and power not otherwise available to you.

There is no more effective tool in the interpretation of your dreams than your journal in which you record your dreams and your interpretations, and your creation of a dream dictionary based on your own analysis of the symbols encountered. This journal is also your *Magical Diary*, for it should contain a record of all your growth and development, and likewise functions as your personal textbook based on all your discoveries. Review your journal often, and you will learn new things from your past experiences with many "Ah-ha!" moments.

PROMOTING QUALITY SLEEP, QUALITY DREAMING, AND QUALITY LIFE

As we've seen, sleep is more than a state of rest—it's a growth and development process as well. It provides a dynamic gateway to the subconscious with its vast wealth of empowering resources. By sleeping and dreaming better, you can tap into those resources to bring new power into your life. Beyond that, sleep can become a gateway to other realms of enlightenment and power. By sleeping and dreaming better, you can access those higher realms and interact with them to empower your life. At a highly practical level, you can enrich your social relationships, accelerate your career progress, and increase your sense of personal well-being. More specifically, you can improve your sex life, reduce negative stress, overcome barriers to your development, and find greater happiness in your daily life.

Fortunately, you can make simple changes in your daily activities that will enrich your total life, to include that important part spent in sleep. Beginning now, you can intervene in ways that will bring new power and abundance into your life. Here are a few examples:

1. **Laugh a little.** Don't take life too seriously. A sense of humor can dissolve blockages and actually generate a more positive situation. Before falling asleep, recall a humorous incident and think about how you feel and felt. A humorous thought can prepare you for sleep by reducing your stress level and generating a more positive mental state.

2. **Expand your thinking, exercise your mental capabilities, and increase your enjoyment of life.** Take time out from the demands of your daily life by stepping back and getting the big picture. You'll find a few moments of strategic withdrawal from a stress situation can improve your coping skills and empower you to work more effectively in difficult situations with difficult people.

3. **Take time to slow down from the headlong rush of life.** Find time to contemplate and reflect. Get in touch with that quiet part of your innermost self. Find ways to slow down the dizzying pace of life.

4. **Get in touch with nature.** Take time to experience the power of nature by interacting with your natural surroundings. A leisurely nature walk among plants and trees can relieve stress and build a powerful sense of well-being. Simply viewing a sunset, the night sky studded with stars, a still lake in the moonlight, or birds in flight can attune the body, mind, and spirit while generating a powerful sense of well-being. When you're unable to interact directly with nature, experiencing nature through visualization can be equally as empowering as firsthand interaction. Visualizing the beauty of nature during the drowsy state preceding sleep is among the best ways known to promote healthful, restful sleep.

5. **Bring variety into your life by adding something new and contrasting.** If you tend to be inflexible or too organized, bring

some spontaneity and open-endedness into your daily activities. If you tend to be too focused on problems and limitations, find ways to exercise your creative side. Take time to think beyond the box. Before falling asleep, you can promote healthful sleep by taking in a deep breath and sensing the possibilities of your life expanding as you exhale slowly.

6. **Establish simple empowerment cues for use in your daily life to replenish your energies and lower your stress level.** For instance, a sip of water from a bedside glass before falling asleep can be a useful cue for promoting healthful sleep and empowering dreams. A sip of water upon awakening can promote recall of your dreams and a better understanding of their relevance. During the drowsy state preceding sleep, you can establish empowering cues for use on demand. Examples are simply turning your head to your right or left to reduce stress, standing or sitting straight to increase mental efficiency and alertness, or visualizing a number or word to generate harmony and balance within.

7. **Exercise your creative powers.** Find ways of tapping into your creative side. Here are a few possibilities: (1) Use word association by first saying a word and then allowing another word to come to mind. Take a few moments to contemplate on the present, past, or future relevance of that word. (2) While reciting the alphabet, spontaneously stop at a certain letter and tell yourself, "This letter is important to me because ..." (3) Clear your mind and allow a colorful image to form. Take a few moments to explore the relevance of the image, particularly its precognitive implications. (4) Think of a personal goal, mentally envelop it in a bright orb, and visualize it floating upward to unite with a higher dimension of power as you sense your connection to that dimension. Each of these exercises can be used during the day as well as immediately before falling asleep to promote healthful sleep and dreaming. They can also be used immediately upon awakening as a good way to start your day.

8. **Connect to your spiritual side.** Develop your capacity to interact with higher spiritual planes and dimensions. Get to know your spirit guides and find ways of interacting with them. They can be sources of enlightenment, protection, inspiration, and strength. In the drowsy state before falling asleep, you can invite a spirit presence to guide your sleep and dream experience. By staying connected to your spiritual side, you become more fully empowered not only spiritually, but mentally and physically as well.

9. **Explore the meaning of your existence.** Develop ways of interacting with your subconscious as a powerhouse of knowledge. Use sleep and dreams as sources of enlightenment, power, and fulfillment. Explore your past and discover its relevance to the present. Commit yourself to the greater good.

10. **Stay positive.** Keep in mind that the best is yet to come. It may sound trite, but it's still true. Commit yourself to developing your potentials to their peaks while helping others. Do what you can now to make the world a better place for present and future generations.

11. **Renew yourself daily.** A major benefit of quality sleeping and dreaming is an empowered state of comprehensive renewal.

CONCLUSION

Conventional wisdom holds that, on average, we develop only a small fraction of our mental potentials. Some estimates place the figure at no more than ten percent overall. Heredity and environment are among the key determining factors in our development, but the most important of all is the choosing self. Through the programs presented in this chapter, you can expand not only your choices but the possibilities as well. You can now choose greatness over mediocrity, success over failure, and abundance over scarcity. You can now take command of your life and make it better for yourself and the world around you.

CHAPTER THREE

INDUCTION AND WORKING WITH THE SUBCONSCIOUS MIND

WHERE DOES THE SUBCONSCIOUS MIND COME FROM?

We are not born with a 'clean slate.' But neither are we born with a fully developed personality preloaded with fully structured Consciousness and a fully defined subconsciousness.

Nor is our consciousness already neatly compartmentalized into conscious, subconscious, and super conscious minds. There are no clearly demarked areas of the brain for each of these three "minds," nor are there established divisions within our consciousness so mapped out.

Nevertheless, we seem to be born with certain 'common seeds' in our consciousness that start developing along approximately the same lines in every child and, as these are "filled in" from experience, they show their common characteristics. They make up parts of the "operating system."

We are, compartmentalized or not, seemingly born with a conscious mind and a subconscious mind, and both are already programmed with an operating system and application programs, and the subconscious mind has various Instincts, Intuitive Knowledge, Memories from Past Lives, and already existing connections with such areas of the subconscious as the Akashic Records, the Archetypes, and such major classifications as Mother, Father, Shadow, Anima, Animus, and even Toys and

Pets. Other ready areas of consciousness include reactions to Pain and Pleasure, Light and Dark, Warmth and Cold, Wet and Dry.

But there are uncommon things that may happen as well, and these become conscious memories of the actual event. Slowly the child learns that certain behaviors when repeated will produce like results. These become rudimentary application programs that eventually progress into methods of communication.

Fresh experiences eventually begin to fall into familiar patterns and some of these are attached to certain of the application programs so that specific actions call up related memories to create a kind of "vocabulary" with which the child expands the range of communication even before speech develops.

During this process, we say that the brain is developing. But we have also to acknowledge the brain is a tool for that area of consciousness we identify as the personality. Behavior is becoming individual and personal. The conscious mind is learning by associating actions with reactions. And the conscious mind is remembering those various associations so it can act with expectation of the reaction. The physical brain is developing as the nonphysical consciousness is learning to use the brain. Despite an increasingly sophisticated educational system, there is still little appreciation of this vital connection and no training specifically related to facilitating it.

It takes a long time for this aspect of the conscious mind to develop—much longer than it does for the child's brain to become an adult brain. And during this time, the conscious mind is also learning and remembering facts and lessons through experience and through education. This process can continue for a lifetime, and even after the physical brain and the body become old and start to deteriorate. The mind may be limited in expression as the brain loses its youthful agility, and then the mind becomes frustrated because it recognizes the age-imposed limitations, showing its superiority and independence over the brain.

But, all along, there are many experiences you've forgotten, and some you have repressed because they were hurtful. They may be forgotten, but they're not gone. They drop from the conscious mind into the subconscious. They are there, but they may not be easily found because there isn't a real structured memory system with organized places, rooms, file folders, or even systematic labeling. You may assume that forgotten or repressed memories are unimportant, but the hurt associated with that repressed memory often lives on, continuing to hurt your feelings, your relationships, and even your body.

The forgotten fact could be important. Like the name of the capital of some distant country might make you the winner of a contest, or forgotten information about a mineral specimen in Montana might literally open a gold mine for you.

Restoring those memories might be a matter of health, or a matter of wealth. And they are there, in your subconscious, and they can be recalled through the technique of self-hypnosis.

The subconscious Mind is like a bank account or trust fund you know little about. When you call upon it with the right code, it delivers principal and profit. But it didn't come with a map or directory of its contents. And, sometimes it doesn't deliver because you didn't ask the right way. It's like a big library catalog that has used different index systems at different times so the wrong input gets wrong results or no results at all.

Where did it all come from? It contains far more 'information' (memories, facts, fears, instructions, etc.) than you've seen in one lifetime. And, that's the point. Many of the subconscious memories do seem to come from previous lives—and, perhaps, not only <u>your</u> past lives! The subconscious mind can be your most important resource and not only for your past memories, or those of your and other past lives, but because it has amazing connections to the entire historic knowledge of humanity and can even probe the unknown.

One name for this is the Akashic Records; another is the collective unconscious. Perhaps they're the same thing or maybe they're different—but the point is that either way you have an amazing resource that most likely you are not using. Accessing it brings self-empowerment. And accessing it is made possible through self-hypnosis.

Expressed another way, self-hypnosis—used properly—is self-empowering.

We're going to teach you how to use self-hypnosis properly, for self-empowerment. But self-empowerment is more than accessing past memories and even all the contents of the collective unconscious. Self-empowerment is the empowering of self, and that self is much more than the familiar self of your personality. This self is the whole person, so much of which is presently beyond your conscious control in the same way so many of those memories are beyond your conscious recall.

PREPARING FOR HYPNOSIS: THE SELF-INDUCTION PROCESS

We start this discussion by recognizing a problem of misrepresentation.

The words "Induction" and "Trance" both suffer the confusion of multiple meanings and various illusions promulgated by their now archaic use in the early history of hypnosis and their inaccurate usage in fantasy fiction and Hollywood movies.

We have already discussed the problem of *Trance* in the Introduction—showing it is not something mysterious imposed by a commanding figure causing the entranced actress (usually) or actor to respond to commands in a slow and monotonous voice, "Yes, Master, I will do as you say." Instead, trance is a word describing a state of consciousness characterized by focused attention and receptivity. It's like really listening without preconceptions and with a real willingness to learn and to believe in with hope for improvement in your life.

Receptivity is the keyword here: the "Subject" (another seemingly goofy word meaning, in hypnosis, the person hypnotized) is voluntarily receptive to suggestions—which may really be new ideas to be considered and hopefully accepted and acted upon. It's as if the "subject" looks you in the eye and earnestly says, "I'm really very interested in what you are saying and can see how it can improve my life. I want to try it. Thank you for making it possible." In other words, you—the subject—understand the benefits to be attained through change of old habits or the addition of new skills and enthusiastically wish to use self-hypnosis to gain those benefits in full acceptance of the technique.

What about this word "Induction?" Some of us associate it with *induction into the military*, where we have given up control of our lives to a hierarchical system unlike our normal world. Other times it may mean induction into a secret society or lodge to which we make a commitment to follow a set of practices or a code of behavior that differs from our normal routines.

We see it in the movies as the commanding hypnotist swings a shiny object before the subject until the eyes close and the subject is in a hypnotic trance. No one can wake him except the hypnotist. Even worse, the hypnotist programs the subject to immediately fall into a trance any time he says a particular word or snaps his fingers. In the fictional world, the subject is no longer in control of his or her own life and is dependent upon an authority figure.

INDUCTION AIDS

But the real world is not the movies. And we know that you can put yourself into a hypnotic state, or trance. Some people do use 'fascination' objects to help them enter a trance state, while others make use of special sound recordings. Neither, of course, is necessary but there is no reason not to make use of them to facilitate the process if you feel a need or desire to do so.

Among the more popular fascination objects are crystal balls (often made of glass), small pocket mirrors, black skrying "magic" mirrors, small pieces of polished black obsidian, spinning swirl discs, flickering candle flames, flickering or whirling lights, and pendulums. Or you can place a device above the head so that one must look up, a position that makes the eyes want to close.

In addition to fascination objects, other induction aids include sound recordings as we've previously mentioned, counting backwards—usually from ten to one—special visualizations including descending elevators or escalators, downward stairs, ocean waves rolling onto the beach, the setting sun descending to and below the horizon, retreating star fields, passing through doorways, scenes in which light is slowly replaced by darkness, etc.

In making the choice of any induction aid, simplicity is best. You don't want to become more interested in the device than in the process; you don't want to be *listening* to music; you don't want to worry about dripping wax or the danger of your candle setting things on fire. The induction aid is intended to help focus your attention inward, not on outward objects.

THE PRINCIPLES OF INDUCTION

Induction is the process that precedes the state of hypnosis, helping the subject to become receptive to new ideas and to change old habits and views. Induction *induces* the state of receptivity. Since we are emphasizing self-hypnosis for self-empowerment, the induction principles are simplified. You wouldn't be hypnotizing yourself if you had not already accepted the concept of hypnosis to bring about desired change and self-improvement and agreed to use it.

Belief and acceptance. One of the values of this book is to affirm with you the importance of both self-empowerment and self-hypnosis in bringing about desired changes and improvements in your life, and the even greater value of putting yourself in charge rather than being dependent upon external authority figures who at best have only secondhand knowledge of your needs and desires and little understanding of your concerns, values, and dreams.

You should read the entire book, and we hope you will read other books from our recommendations. We want you to believe in your own power and your own authority to take command of your life. Self-empowerment is a way of life: a belief in Self (big "S") and a belief in continued evolution and personal growth. We want you to expand beyond your present artificial limitations and become the whole person you are in potential.

Hypnosis is a science, but there is nothing difficult to learning it. Like any applied science, using hypnosis is an art that is personal to the user. The principles of induction are easy to understand and apply, and you will learn to adapt them in making them a normal part of your life. The use of self-hypnosis should become as constant to you as any other positive habit.

Security and confidence. It's up to you to set a location and situation that is secure against disturbance and disruption. Nearly any room with closed doors and windows will do, turning off the telephone and other appliances that could interrupt your session, and leaving instructions—if necessary—that you are not to be disturbed for an hour or other time period. As to confidence—of course you have confidence in yourself. You have no better friend, no better guardian, and no finer guide than yourself. If you feel the need for some form of psychic self-defense, we will provide for that as an option in your own induction process.

Relaxed Body and Calm Mind. You are your own worst enemy and your own best friend. You are in charge of your own body and mind and it is you who can unstress your body and calm the chatter of your mind. Put aside any concerns; think 'blankly' free of wants, desires, worries; don't even think of your goals during this phase. Instruct yourself to hear only your inner voice unless there is a real emergency. (Your inner voice is exactly that: do not speak words, do not even mouth the words, but learn to hear the words in your head as if they were spoken in your own strong voice.)

Learn to think without words; instead think with feelings.

As you breathe, feel yourself doing what you would say with words—such as 'sinking deeper and deeper.' Feel that you are entering into your subconsciousness where you have the power to bring your goals into manifestation. Know that your subconsciousness knows no barriers except those that you, in innocence and ignorance, or fear, self-impose. We will give you specific steps to cleanse the slate.

---

*This relaxation phase is extremely important to the success of the entire program, and should be continued for approximately 15 minutes, and repeated daily! Deep relaxation of body and mind "helps your body and mind to reset and re-center themselves, to normalize physiological processes and to generally restore you at every level of your being."**

* Roger A. Straus, *Creative Self-Hypnosis* (New York: Prentice-Hall, 1989, New York), 102. The included audio CD facilitates this easily.

The Right Time. It is not your goal to fall asleep; hence it is important that you do not conduct your self-hypnosis sessions when you are fatigued and ready for sleep. Sure, it is wonderful to go to sleep after the session, but do not use self-hypnosis to fall asleep unless your problem is insomnia. For this reason, it is preferable to conduct your session seated in a chair rather than lying in bed. A recliner may be acceptable provided you are not too "laid back."

For many people the better times may be early morning or early evening. You want to be alert but not ready to hit a home run or feel disturbed by the morning or evening news. "Calm" and "alert" are your keywords in choosing the time.

THE KEY STEPS IN THE INDUCTION PROCESS

Preparation

Identify. Before selecting a problem or goal for your self-hypnosis intervention, it is important that you identify what it is that you really want. Go into your general meditation procedure and ask to see yourself as you want to be. Don't be in a hurry, and don't presume that you already know the important problems or goals. Ask questions and let your subconscious give you some answers. If there are not immediate responses, ask yourself questions about the self-image you want to see in relation to health, appearance, career, relationships, family, etc. Find two or three important self-images expressing particular problems or goals, and decide which the most important one now is, and keep the rest for later.

The Problem. Knowing what you really want, select a problem to resolve or a goal for action, such as losing weight. Make your goal reasonable. If it is too grand, you may lose confidence in its attainment. There should be no doubt in your mind that it can be done. If necessary, break a larger goal down into a series of logical shorter goals, but be careful not to minimize the process. If you weigh 300 pounds, losing 100 pounds is not too large a goal. If you weigh 150 pounds, 25 pounds might be just right.

It is better to focus on a single goal at a time, or you can add two or three closely related sub-goals to it. Make sure that the sub-goals support the major goal.

Write it down. Write down your reasons for taking action. Build a solid case, and show the benefits. Following our example of weight loss, it might be for health reasons or for appearance. Be specific and justify the program. For most people, a present weight of 300 pounds is hard on the heart, on the knees, on the pancreas, etc. It may also be difficult to find attractive clothing. That much weight is probably fatiguing. So much weight may affect your sleep, even causing sleep apnea. And if your doctor or your spouse is telling you to lose weight, write that down as well. Convince yourself of the desirability of your goal.

Analyze the Challenge. You have a problem, and you know the reasons to make the change. But, if that was all there was to it you would have solved the problem long ago. You have to ask yourself why it is that you still have the problem, in this example, overweight. Deep inside, in your subconscious, there are reasons you overeat despite your desire to be physically fit and attractive. Why do you do something that *rationally* you know that you should not?

Be honest in digging up those answers; some of them may be embarrassing; some of them may be hurtful—but it's important to understand the origins of the problem in order to change from old to new. The reasons for change outweigh the old reasons that caused the problem, but you have to see them for what they are—old, tired illusions.

Write them down right next to the reasons to change, and see how the new cancel out the old.

Write your expectations. Write down your expectations for results. Look into the future and see yourself as you want to be, and see all that it involves. In regard to the example weight problem, are there particular factors that you need to acknowledge as difficulties to be overcome?

Write the I AM sentence. Write a short, single sentence starting with "I AM" that expresses the successful outcome of the self-hypnosis you are about to undertake. An example would be: "I AM slim." Always keep the "I AM" in capital letters. This is a statement of the goal accomplished, of the new reality that has replaced the old.

Memorize it. Say it to yourself in a way that *feels* meaningful and powerful. Speak the words out loud and listen to them, and memorize the sound, the inflection, and the feeling. Then say it silently while hearing it in your head with the same feelings as when spoken out loud. Say it with energy. Say it with certainty that it already is. You will say it silently with your inner voice.

Visualize it. Close your eyes and visualize the sentence in White Letters against a black background. As you see it, speak the sentence with your inner voice.

See it now. Build a picture of the future in which your problem is resolved, your goal attained. Remember: you are leaving the old reality behind and see yourself already living in the new reality. See it, feel it, think it, believe it—you are there now. You are in the new reality. Write it down.

This is another extremely important part of the process, and why daily repetition is vital. The audio CD facilitates this for you, but you still must understand the need and apply the technique.

Once is not enough. To make a new reality for yourself you have to experience it over and over. This goes for new realities inside your mind and also in the outside world. Until experience is reinforced, and until imaginary experience is rekindled, again and again, it will not seem real to you; you will not respond to the experience as real and you won't be able to work with it.

At the same time, if you are trying to break out of the ordinary—including the ordinary for yourself—you are fighting the resistance of the whole world. It is going to gnaw at your inner realities, try to erode them away into more of the same. Your best defensive weapon, perhaps your only weapon, is to be stubborn and to keep on imagining over your chosen reality.*

* Straus, 1989, 102.

Meditation

Comfort and Security. Make yourself comfortable and arrange things so you will not be disturbed except for a genuine emergency. Sit either upright or partially reclining, but do not lie down unless that's a physical necessity for you. Dim the lights to a comfortable level. It is preferable that you do not have incense burning or background music or a soundtrack, except as will be discussed later. You want to avoid the distraction that these otherwise niceties can provide.

Relaxation. Do your regular relaxation to enter into meditation. One very powerful procedure is called "Tension and Release," made up of the following steps:

Tense all muscles. Take a deep breath and hold it while tensing all your muscles, from head to toe, including the facial muscles. Feel the muscle contraction in your jaw, around your eyes, even around your ears, feel it in your neck and shoulders, chest and arms, make fists, feel the contraction in your chest, abdomen, groin, upper thighs, knees, and calves, and point your toes. Hold your body with all the muscles in deep tensions until you have to let your breath out, and then relax as you breathe out completely, letting go of all tension, mind chatter, and emotional concerns.

An alternative is called 'fractional relaxation' where you tense first your toes and then release, then your foot and release, progressing up the body all the way to the scalp. After you've done it a few times, you will be amazed at how fast and how completely you will relax the whole body.

Breathe fully and regularly. Breathe deeply, in and out, in and out, again and again. Feel and see the oxygen-rich air filled with life energy filling your lungs and spreading throughout your body. Then as you exhale, feel and see the out-breath carrying away waste products. Your body feels refreshed, healed, and deeply relaxed. Feel yourself fully cleansed physically and mentally.

Finding the center. Continue the regular breathing, continue feeling cleansed and relaxed, and a moment will come when you feel yourself experiencing an inner awakening, opening like a flower into full receptivity. Continue enjoying this blissful state, feeling calmness, vitality, peacefulness, and strength, ready to receive your self-instruction.

See and Hear your I AM sentence. When ready, see your memorized sentence in white letters against a black background in your Mind's Eye. Hold that vision for about two minutes (Do not count seconds and do not open your eyes to check the actual time. Just do it until you feel satisfied) while silently saying the sentence slowly with feeling and inflection. Listen to your inner voice and hear it with your inner ears so it seems just as if you were hearing it aloud.

Image or Symbol. Now, silently ask your subconscious mind to produce a simple image or symbol to fully represent that sentence. If nothing comes to you, repeat daily until it does. (There is a difference between an image and a symbol. A symbol is usually something already existing, often a three-dimensional object, with particular ideas and energies associated with it. Those ideas and energies must be in harmony with your I AM sentence to work effectively for you. An image is usually a simple picture or visual pattern created by your subconscious to work with your "I AM" sentence.) Memorize it, and draw it—no matter what your artistic skills are.

Memorize it. See your image or symbol in the same mental scene as your "I AM" sentence. Know that you now have the power to make your dream come true, the power to realize your goal, the power to make it your new reality replacing the old reality.

The New Reality. Remember that we are not merely leaving old habits behind but an old reality and replacing it with a new reality that is your own. Think about yourself in the future that will be after you have solved your problem, after you have fulfilled your goal. See yourself in this new reality as if it has already happened. Make this your future NOW. Feel yourself in the new reality, repeat your vision of the image and your "I AM" sentence together, and hear your inner voice say it. Tie it all together so any time you repeat the sentence in your mind, you know that what is accomplished in the Inner World is manifesting in the physical world, and that your Body, Mind and Spirit are working together to bring this about.

PSYCHIC SELF-DEFENSE AND A STRONG AURA

Psychic self-defense is based on two simple principles: (1) self-confidence and (2) a strongly visualized aura.

Self-empowerment will increase your self-confidence, but what do we really mean by 'confidence in self?' Certainly it is not a false belief that you can't be hurt in accidents or by physical weapons. The dictionary definition is redundant: "confidence in yourself and your own abilities." The thesaurus goes a little further and compares it to self-assurance, self-possession, poise.

What do we mean when we say that President Obama exhibits lots of self-confidence? Yes, he believes in his message to the people, he believes in his ability as a leader, he is confident that he can fulfill the obligations of his office and negotiate from a position of strength and 'rightness.' He does not doubt his abilities to meet challenges and his skills in working with people.

Perhaps more than anything else, self-confidence means that you know your self and what your skills and limitations actually are. It means you are confident within a defined sphere of operations based on knowledge and understanding of who you are.

In truth, everything we do successfully starts with knowledge of self, and everything we do in self-improvement starts with self-understanding. With self-knowledge we can build our lives with confidence, i.e., with self-confidence. So, self-defense starts with self-knowledge—you do not put yourself in a place of danger without full awareness of the challenges and you do so with a full understanding of what must be done to protect yourself in these circumstances.

Your aura is somewhat different. You have more than a physical body: in the whole person you are, you have etheric, astral, mental, and spiritual bodies all interconnected through various energy systems and conduits. Essentially, however, we can group those beyond the physical under the collective name of your "psychic body."

Every body is a combination of substance and energy, and because of this, every living body is radiant. Your body is surrounded by a radiance called an "aura." Because your psychic body responds to thought and emotion, you can deliberately shape and strengthen its outer surface to act as a protective shield that bounces any kind of psychic attack off the surface and returns it to the sender.

Let's step back for just a moment. Good defense starts not with offense but with *intelligence* about your potential enemy. Do you really know of anyone 'out to get you'? Self-confidence and a strong aura will often deter common physical attacks. Now, do you know of anyone who could wish you psychic harm, and who has the skill and power to do so? Probably not—especially in recognition that such an attack will be reflected back to the sender multiplied three-fold in strength.

When you are in a position of receptivity, you are open to the psychic world. Some people believe there are negative entities eager to attack and possess the human soul. We've never encountered such beings, but the truth is that your soul is not part of your psychic body, per se. It's "above" it and no entity can harm or possess it.

Nevertheless, just as physical fitness is desirable, so is psychic fitness. And just as there are exercises to improve your physical fitness, so are there exercises to strengthen your aura. Remember that your aura responds to thought and emotion.

Go through your preliminary regimen of physical relaxation and mental and emotional calmness. While breathing deeply and regularly, without any strain, picture that your in-breath is filled with bright life energy, and on the out-breath this energy spreads throughout your body. After a half-dozen such energy-laden breaths, on the out-breath visualize your aura and see it becoming brighter and brighter. When it is very radiant, further visualize a radiant outer surface and know that it will reflect any kind of psychic or spiritual negativity. Hold that image for a few moments and know that it is always there, no matter how receptive you are to psychic and spiritual communications.

That's all that is needed, but we will include a guided aura-strengthening exercise in your guided program on the accompanying audio CD.

SELF-HYPNOSIS AND THE SPECIAL AUDIO CD

Utilizing the above principles of induction, you can incorporate your goals into your own dynamic, self-empowering self-hypnosis programs for virtually any need. You have the power and now you have the knowledge. It requires thoughtful planning and determined practice, but you now see how to directly involve the most powerful assets you have—your subconscious mind with your conscious rational mind—to take control of your life on your own terms.

THE I AM PRINCIPLE OF SUGGESTIONS

It probably is obvious to all our readers, but it is such an important point that it needs to be emphatically stated: *Since we are involved with self-hypnosis, the word "you" is banned from all dialogue.* And we nearly as emphatically urge that no dialogue used in self-hypnosis refer to yourself as if objectively by name. In other words, never address yourself in self-hypnosis by your name, social security number, or other public identity.

Yes, our names are our public identity, but they are not nearly as affirmative as our personal identity. Only one word identifies the person involved in self-hypnosis and that person is known only as "I."

All internal dialogue, all hypnotic suggestions, all affirmations are to be stated in the first person "I."

A second point that must be made is that all dialogue and imagery is stated and seen in the present tense and circumstance. "I AM here now" is the basis for all the statements made to yourself during induction, receptive state, and afterwards. A third point is to keep these statements simple.

A statement like "I AM slim" is personal, concise, and entirely present tense. Rather than self-deceptive or delusional, it is a picture of your goal accomplished. That is the new reality that has replaced the old reality. You cannot occupy two realities at the same time, and a statement like "I AM *becoming slimmer*" is ambiguous and defeating. To mobilize your power of creative thought, *you have to see things as you want them to be and see yourself in that new reality.* See it completely and see it like a movie with you living that new reality in everyday detail.

PSYCHOMETRY AND ASTRAL GATEWAYS

Self-hypnosis can be used in various ways. Mostly we think in terms of replacing old realities with new. We get rid of old bad habits and adopt a new life style that accomplishes goals of health, wealth, and purpose. But self-hypnosis can also be used to tap into a wealth of knowledge via focus on specific symbols.

We will develop this theme further in chapter six with discussion of actual applications of astral techniques, but here we include induction using symbols rich in associations that open specific repositories of the subconscious mind. The same technique can be used to access both personal memories and memories associated with such personal objects as Grandfather's watch.

"Psychometry" is the word associated with accessing memories and impressions related to an object, while "skrying" is used in relationship to symbols such as Tarot Cards, the Runes, I Ching Hexagrams, Yantras, and also the use of particular objects as tools to access areas of knowledge.

The induction process is the same as previously outlined up to the point at which you would assert your I AM statements and Images of personal goals. In their place, you will instead use these richly "pre-loaded" symbols that will bring you into contact with specific archetypes (powerful images representing areas of human experience—such as Mother, Priest, Lover, Sun, Moon, Warrior, Priestess, etc.) or with specific energies and currents that act as switches that stir energy responses in the physical and psychic bodies.

In both cases, skrying moves consciousness from one thing to another, triggering new inner experiences and tapping new knowledge. It becomes a whole program of learning controlled by the choice of symbols and the sequences with which they are used.

From an observer's viewpoint, it would be described as meditation upon the object, sometimes brought up and pressed to the forehead as if to the "third" or psychic eye, and other times with the objects placed in patterns on the surface before the user.

Objectless Meditation

Just as that point in the induction process before you would interject your I AM affirmations can be used for skrying and psychometry with objects, it can be used in "open-minded" meditation. Here the goal is communication—perhaps with spirits, perhaps with elemental entities, perhaps with advanced beings, perhaps with elements of your own subconsciousness. Or from your superconsciousness.

You'll never know who's talking unless you're listening.

All of this will be discussed in greater detail in later chapters. The point of bringing them up now is to show you the potential of the meditative consciousness.

CHAPTER FOUR

Scripts and Dialogues: Specific Suggestions for Different Applications

YOU WERE BORN TO BE GREAT!

Self-Empowerment is the Transforming Next Step.

All your life, you have essentially been molded and trained by others. You were born with a genetic composition reflecting not only your parents, grandparents, and all who have gone before, and then you were trained and programmed first by your parents and other caregivers, then by a slowly expanding social environment starting mostly with that television set filled with brightly colored cartoons.

With each birthday, your social world expanded outward, with more and more guidance, training, modeling, and then education from outside the family unit. And the more the external influence, the more pressure there was for conformity to various abstract ideals—in behavior, clothing, activities, dating, summer jobs, college, getting a job, settling down, marriage, starting a family, buying a home, applying for a mortgage, raising your children, and repeating all that went before with them.

All along, other external factors may have increased the pressures to conformity, including educational and professional requirements, the military, job expectations, the social life of your friends and neighbors, and on and on. In all that we do, we are in *transition* to new situations that are mostly controlled by others.

It's not that there was or is anything bad about this, it's just the fact that you are not really used to *shaping your own destiny* or even

69

understanding who you are. It's even a difficult concept to think that you might not know much about yourself or that you might want and can actually have more control over your life. After all, dependence is part of childhood, but has *adulthood really brought independence?*

And, what does independence mean? Doesn't the 'system' for the most part take care of you? *What about those areas where it fails you— an economy that goes into recession, international situations that lead to war, foods that make you obese, cars bigger than you need, houses you can't afford, drugs that hurt you, security that fails to protect you, and the mistakes other people make for which you become the victim?*

Then, in contrast, there is the inner world of spirit and those innate powers that you need to understand and develop to become the whole person you were born to be.

Thankfully, it is no longer a matter of course to assume that you smoke cigarettes, but let's just assume you are a smoker. Realize that you became a smoker through a multiplicity of external influences— modeling from your peers, being influenced by celebrities smoking, by advertisements making smoking exciting and glamorous, even sexy, and so on. And, then, of course, you became addicted—another external influence. Now, let's assume you looked at the situation and decided you didn't like what you saw. You understood how you were manipulated to adopt a habit both costly and unhealthy. Then you decide you want to change, you want to take charge of your life and shape your own destiny.

You want to be *self-empowered,* but you find it difficult. The chemical addiction and the habit of many years of shaking out a cigarette when you want to relax and think something over are fighting your desire to change. Until you can overcome these, you are not in charge of your own life. You lack power over your destiny. You know smoking is not good for you, but you can't stop. It's as if you are a slave to a sadistic devil gleefully cracking the whip.

What a grim situation that is!

SELF-EMPOWERMENT IS A MATTER OF CHOICE

Smoking is just one example; because you know that many people are no longer smokers, you do know that it is possible to stop and you can even see that eliminating some of the external conditioning factors makes it easier. There are many other examples. But let's just assume that you've 'beat the habit' and now see more clearly that *you can make positive changes in your life.* There's more to life than the system provides. There's more security in life when you understand what's going on. There's more opportunity in life when you can make your own intelligent choices.

That's right: *you can take charge of your life.* You can 'transition' from others controlling your life to a life of self-control and self-empowerment—making decisions for your own self and now accomplishing those actual changes away from old behavior and habits, and choosing new programs of health and betterment, and then developing your innate powers to function for your greater growth and abilities. It may sound grandiose but the truth is that you were born to be great, you were born to become more than you are, but *it can only happen when you actually do it for your self.*

SELF-EMPOWERMENT IS DYNAMIC

Self-empowerment as a growth process exists in a dynamic continuum that's constantly receptive to your interaction. The self-empowerment scripts presented in this chapter are designed to put you in command of that continuum and to demonstrate how you can write your own scripts at will. Each script is based on the twofold concept:

1. Vast sources of power exist both within yourself and externally to yourself—all of which are available to you, and

2. You can discover those resources and use them to empower and enrich your life.

Activating your dormant potentials, achieving your personal goals, discovering your personal spirit guides, and interacting with higher spiritual planes are all possible through the scripts presented here. By taking command, you are constantly becoming more than you are. You are growing into becoming a self-empowered whole person in charge of your own destiny.

A major goal of self-empowerment scripts, however, is not only to draw forth power, but equally as important, *to generate a deeply meaningful interaction within the self.* Every part of your being is related. Through relevant self-empowerment scripts, you will discover new ways of balancing and attuning the mind, body, and spirit to result in a more fully empowered state that gives new meaning to your existence as an evolving soul.

Self-empowerment scripts recognize the critical importance of the messages we send to ourselves through a variety of channels that include not only our thoughts and verbal expressions but also our emotions, aspirations, perceptions, and attitudes—in other words, every aspect of our being.

THE IMPORTANCE OF SELF-DIALOGUE

At its best, positive self-dialogue is not only self-empowering, it is also self-validating. Such affirmations as *I am a person of intrinsic worth* and *Success is my destiny* can shape and sustain a powerful self-image that is the essential foundation for personal growth and success.

While positive self-dialogue strengthens and validates the self system, negative self-dialogue weakens it. Such negative messages as *I'm a failure; my future is bleak; my feelings are unimportant* and so forth are at once self-devaluing and self-disempowering. They discredit the self and deprive it of its most powerful resource—the awareness of personal dignity and worth. Fortunately, positive dialogue consistently overpowers negative dialogue—they cannot coexist. Nothing more effectively extinguishes the disempowering effects of negative dialogue than positive affirmations of personal worth.

THE POWER OF IMAGES OF ACCOMPLISHMENT

The success of self-empowerment scripts depends largely on positive, goal-related dialogue accompanied by related visualization. When combined with appropriate visualization, the power of positive dialogue increases many times over. While stating your goals in positive terms is important, visualizing yourself having achieved them and experiencing the emotional rewards of success multiplies beyond measure the power of dialogue. In addition, you can use simple symbolism to add substance to goals related to your subconscious potentials. For instance, visualizing your goals as pebbles dropped into the pool of your subconscious can effectively connect you to the inner resources required for your complete success.

This combination of dialogue and imagery can be especially effective in activating your dormant psychic potentials, including ESP and PK. Along another line, for goals related to rejuvenation and health, imagining yourself diving into a pool of healthful, rejuvenating energy can dramatically increase the effectiveness of suggestions alone. Yet another highly effective approach uses visualization of bright rays of light that connect you to the highest planes of power, as we'll later see. When followed with positive affirmations of complete success, the use of goal-related dialogue and visualization becomes even more powerful.

It's not unusual for important goal-related images to spontaneously emerge at any stage of a given script. You can facilitate that process early on by simply stating your goal and then pausing long enough for important images to form in your mind. As you move slowly from stage to stage throughout the script, other relevant images will often unfold, at times with profound empowerment potential. Keep in mind that *the most powerful images are those that emerge naturally from within.*

The scripts that follow can be used effectively with any appropriate self-hypnosis induction program. Each script, however, is flexible and can be applied with equal effectiveness under a variety of other conditions, such as meditation, relaxation, thoughtful repose, and the drowsy state preceding sleep. Given sufficient previous practice, you may find that applying a familiar script immediately upon awakening can also be highly effective. The specific dialogue, affirmations, visualizations, and post-script cues as detailed in each script are offered as examples or guidelines which can be easily revised to fit your individual preferences and style. You may find that the most effective scripts are those you adapt or modify while retaining their essential elements.

Before applying a selected script, it's important to first become familiar with the full script by reviewing each step carefully. Once you have an overview of the script and are comfortable with it, set aside approximately thirty minutes to implement it in a quiet, relaxed setting. You'll find that repeated practice will increase the effectiveness of each script.

SCRIPT 1: DEVELOPING YOUR ESP AND PK POTENTIALS

This script is based on the premise that psychic potentials exist in everyone. Through appropriate practice and experience, you can develop those potentials and apply them to achieve your goals and enrich your life. You can develop your extrasensory perception (ESP) powers that include *telepathy* or the ability to communicate mentally with others, *precognition* or the ability to perceive future events, and *clairvoyance* or the ability to mentally perceive conditions and distant events. You can develop your *psychokinetic* (PK) powers or your ability to mentally influence happenings and processes. Through the script that follows, you can establish the essential conditions required to exercise each of these potentials and thus promote their full development.

Step 1. Goal Statement. Begin the script by stating in your own words your goal of developing your ESP and PK potentials. Record your goal statement in your journal.

Step 2. Focused Attention and Receptivity. Induce a state of focused attention and receptivity to suggestion, either through self-hypnosis or, if you prefer, through the use of a preferred meditation or deep relaxation program. Yet another highly effective option is the use of the drowsy state preceding sleep.

Step 3. Self-Empowerment Dialogue. While in the deeply receptive state, initiate positive self-dialogue related to your stated goal. Here are a few examples.

I am psychic by nature.

My psychic potentials are essential to my personal evolvement. They are basic to my mental, physical, and spiritual existence.

I am committed to developing my ESP and PK powers to their peaks.

I will find ways of using my ESP and PK powers to enrich my life.

By embracing my ESP powers, I expand the scope of my existence and give new meaning to my life.

Day by day, I will use my psychic powers to enrich my life and bring forth desired change.

At this point, you may wish to present in your own words additional dialogue specific to your personal goals and present life situation. Examples include dialogue related to social relationships, career success, problem solving, and personal improvement, to mention but a few. Such dialogue focuses your self-empowerment program to the Here and Now.

Step 4. Visualization. As you remain in the deeply focused and receptive state, draw and visualize a Triangle of Light* as a channel through which to experience your psychic powers. By centering your attention on the bright space within the triangle, you will become empowered to send and receive telepathic messages, allow images of precognitive significance to emerge, and view distant realities, both material and spiritual. You can use the triangle as a framework for exercising your PK power to influence events and conditions, including internal biological functions related to better health and wellness. Managing pain, promoting healing, and stimulating rejuvenation are all available to you through the Triangle of Light.

Step 5. Affirmation. Affirm in your own words that you are now empowered to exercise your psychic powers at will. Further affirm that you will use your ESP and PK powers to promote your personal evolvement while contributing to the good of others.

---

* The Triangle of Light is simply an equilateral triangle of light that you create in your imagination as *you draw it with the index finger of your stronger hand.* The physical act of drawing it gives 'substance' to the visualization.

Step 6. Post-script Cue. Affirm that by simply visualizing the Triangle of Light, you will become empowered at any moment to activate the full effects of this script. This mental cue is applicable to any situation and its results are instant.

Step 7. Exit and Conclusion. Give yourself permission to exit the trance or other receptive state. End the script by taking a few moments to reflect on the relevance of this experience to your present life situation. You will further enable it by recording the entire experience in your journal.

You can accelerate the development of your ESP and PK skills through repeated use of this script along with practice in a variety of real-life situations. For instance, you can fine-tune your telepathic skills by working with others in sending and receiving telepathic messages. You can exercise your precognitive skills by visualizing future happenings, to include events ranging from personal relevance to widespread global significance. You can exercise your clairvoyant skills by such activities as locating a lost article or identifying the contents of a package before opening it. You can practice your PK ability by such exercises as bringing a stationary object, such as a crumpled piece of paper, into motion. Use your creative powers to design your own practice exercises. Keep a journal of your progress.

With practice, you will note rapid development of your psychic skills along with such spin-off benefits as increased feelings of competency and overall enrichment in the quality of your life. Clearly, developing your psychic powers is well worth your time and effort.

SCRIPT 2: INTERACTING WITH SPIRIT GUIDES

This script is based on the twofold concept that the spirit dimension does exists and that you, as a spirit being, can interact with it. This script recognizes that you are not only mind and body but also spirit. Without the spirit, the mind and body would not exist. Even the physical universe at large is sustained by the spiritual force that underlies it.

This script recognizes that as a soul being, your existence is forever—from everlasting to everlasting. All things physical have a beginning and therefore an end. Difficult though it may be to comprehend, you as a soul existed forever before your first lifetime and you will exist forever beyond your last. Within that endless spectrum, you are inextricably linked to the spirit realm. You came from that realm, and you will return to it. Rather than a cold, distant, inaccessible realm, it is a present though a nonphysical dimension of power that is available to you at any moment. As a soul, you are in fact integrally connected to it.

Through your interactions with that dimension, you can become increasingly empowered to fulfill the basic purpose of your existence in this physical realm—to learn and grow while, at the same time, helping others and contributing to a better world. Spirit guides from the spirit realm are constantly poised to promote your fulfillment of that all-important purpose. This script is designed to promote empowering interactions with those spirit guides.

(This script makes no presumptions about the form that your Spirit Guide may assume in your consciousness, and neither should you. Spirit is multidimensional and nondimensional. Your Guide will manifest as most beneficial to your needs—as a wise person, a loving animal, an angelic being, or a mere presence. You may experience your guide in vision, as a voice, or in just knowing. There may be dialogue or there may just be a flash of knowledge. Spirit knows no boundaries and your spirit, too, is without bounds.)

Step 1. Goal Statement. Begin the script by stating in your own words your goal of interacting with spirit guides. You may wish to include other specific goals related to that interaction, such as solving a particular personal problem, achieving career success, building self-esteem, or coping with a difficult life situation. Record your goal statement in your journal.

Step 2. Focused Attention and Receptivity. Induce a state of focused attention and receptivity to suggestion, either through self-hypnosis or another preferred option, such as meditation, deep relaxation, or the drowsy state preceding sleep.

Step 3. Self-Empowerment Dialogue. While in the deeply receptive state, initiate positive self-dialogue related to your stated goal. Here are a few examples:

I am more than mind and body, I am also spirit—the essential essence of my existence.

As a spirit being, I am intimately connected to the spirit realm and its wealth of empowerment resources.

I am at this moment empowered to engage the spirit realm and interact with spirit guides that make up that bright dimension.

My interactions with the spirit realm are essential to my growth as an evolving soul.

Step 4. Visualization. As you remain in the deeply focused and receptive state, visualize a beam of light connecting you to the spirit realm as a glowing dimension of unparalleled beauty. Rather than some distant, untouchable realm, think of it as spiritually present with spirit guides in clear view. Should you decide to do so, you can even reach out and touch that realm and embrace its spirit guides.

Step 5. Affirmation. Affirm your resolve to engage in an ongoing interaction with your personal spirit guides as sources of enlightenment, support, and fulfillment. As you continue the interaction, you can again state your personal goals and invite the support of spirit guides in achieving them. (At this step, a particular guide will sometimes come forward, and its name will become known.)

Step 6. Post-script Cue. Affirm that by simply visualizing the bright beam of light connecting you to the spirit dimension, you can instantly generate an interaction with your spirit guide(s) and activate the full empowering effects of this script.

Step 7. Exit and Conclusion. End the script by giving yourself permission to exit the trance or other receptive state. Take as long as you need to reflect on the experience and its empowering relevance.

The script now complete, reaffirm in your own words the spiritual essence of your existence and the supremacy of the spiritual over the physical. Express your appreciation of the guiding presence you came to know through this script. Take time to enjoy that presence as a source of comfort, power, and joy. Record the experience in your journal.

SCRIPT 3: DEVELOPING YOUR MEDIUMISTIC POTENTIALS

The mediumistic potential is the capacity to directly communicate with entities in the spirit realm. The skilled medium is anyone who has developed that potential and applies it, often to initiate communication with a departed relative or friend. At another level, the skill can be applied to initiate interactions with highly advanced spirit beings who can be important sources of spiritual enlightenment and knowledge.

This script is based on the premise that the mediumistic potential exists to some degree in everyone. The best medium is, in fact, already a part of your innermost self. Through this script, that personal medium can become an invaluable source of spiritual insight and personal power. Mediumistic communications that utilize that inner medium can increase your feelings of self-worth, promote inner balance and attunement, and inspire you to reach your highest peak of spiritual growth. Here's the script.

Step 1. Goal Statement. Formulate your goal of developing your mediumistic potentials and using them to empower your life. In stating your goal, you may wish to specify the discovery of advanced spirit teachers who will facilitate your mediumistic development. Record your goal statement in your journal.

Step 2. Focused Attention and Receptivity. Induce a state of focused attention and receptivity to suggestion, either through self-hypnosis or some other referred option, such as meditation, deep relaxation, or the drowsy state preceding sleep.

Step 3. Self-Empowerment Dialogue. While in the deeply focused and receptive state, initiate positive self-dialogue related to the development and application of your mediumistic potentials. Here are a few examples:

I am a spiritual being, and my destiny is spiritual evolvement.

By interacting with the spirit dimension, I am fulfilling that destiny and bringing deeper meaning into my life.

By developing my mediumistic powers, I am becoming empowered to communicate and interact with spirit entities existing in the spirit dimension.

My mediumistic interactions are critical to my understanding of myself and my destiny.

I am committed to using my mediumistic powers to accelerate my spiritual evolvement while contributing to the greater good.

Step 4. Visualization. Visualize a gateway to the spirit realm and imagine yourself opening it to reveal a dimension of indescribable beauty. Sense the peace and harmony flowing from that dimension permeating your total being. Notice the presence of others beyond the gate and the bright glow enveloping them. At this point, you may recognize certain departed loved ones, friends, and familiar spirit guides who have been with you in the past. Give yourself permission to communicate and interact with them. You will notice that beings on the other side can come and go through the gateway to interact with souls on this side. Clearly, it's a spiritual gateway of interaction, not separation. You too can briefly slip through that gate to interact with the spirit realm, should you decide to do so. Adding to the beauty of the spirit realm is the presence of animals and plant life—could it be heaven without them? To conclude this step, visualize yourself closing the gateway, thus ending your mediumistic interaction with the other side.

Step 5. Affirmation. Affirm your strong commitment to use your mediumistic powers to gain knowledge of spiritual relevance and use it as needed to promote your spiritual evolvement while contributing to the higher good.

Step 6. Post-script Cue. Give yourself the post-script cue that you can at any moment activate your mediumistic powers by simply visualizing the gateway to the spirit realm and yourself opening it.

Step 7. Exit and Conclusion. Conclude this script by giving yourself permission to exit the trance or other receptive state. Take time to reflect on the information gained during the experience and your sense of spiritual empowerment. Record your experience.

This script opens an exciting gateway to the spirit realm as an unlimited source of power and knowledge. Through repeated practice of the script, you will fine-tune your ability to use your mediumistic powers. You will discover ways of applying them at will to increase your understanding of your present and future existence. You will discover that the other side is a rich dimension of continued growth and fulfillment. You will see your present life as filled with wondrous opportunities for growth and fulfillment. You will see death, not as a sad closing of a door, but as a marvelous gateway to another dimension filled with limitless possibilities.

SCRIPT 4: DISCOVERING HIGHER PLANES OF POWER

The script is based on the premise that the spirit dimension consists of not only spirit beings but also many planes, each of a different power. Through this script, you will discover ways of interacting with different planes and accessing their unique powers. You will discover that the color of a given plane provides a valuable guide to its power attribute.

Interestingly, the significance of color in the spirit realm is not unlike that associated with the human aura. Radiant green, for instance, in the human and the spirit realm alike, is typically associated with healing, clear blue with serenity, and yellow with intelligence, to list but a few. Our lab studies found that through this script, *you can actually introduce a new color and the power it signifies into your aura by interacting with a higher plane of that color.* That finding suggests that higher planes are not simply lifeless or dormant repositories of color, but rather dynamic life-force energies that are readily accessible to each of us to enrich and empower our lives. Here's the script.

Step 1. Goal Statement. State in your own words your goal of discovering higher planes of power and interacting with them to access their wide-ranging powers. You may wish to address specific concerns related to your present life situation, such as social relationships, finances, health and fitness, academic or career success, and rejuvenation, to mention but a few. Record your goal statement in your journal.

Step 2. Focused Attention and Receptivity. Induce a state of focused attention and receptivity to suggestion, either through self-hypnosis or, if you prefer, through the use of a preferred meditation or deep relaxation program. Yet another highly effective option is the use of the drowsy state preceding sleep. For this script, it is important to relax your hands either in your lap or to your sides with the palms turned upward.

Step 2. Self-Empowerment Dialogue. While in the deeply focused and receptive state, initiate positive self-dialogue related to your goal of discovering and interacting with higher planes of power. Here are a few examples:

Life-force energy is essential to my existence as an evolving soul.

The higher planes of life-force energy are constantly available to me and receptive to my interest and interactions.

I am fully committed to developing my capacity to interact with higher planes of power.

By interacting with higher planes of power, I can achieve even my most difficult goals.

I am enriched mentally, physically, and spiritually through my interactions with higher planes of power.

Balance, attunement, and success are now available to me through my interactions with higher planes of power.

Note: You may wish at this point to include highly specific dialogue related to particular personal goals, such as better health, stress control, problem solving, or breaking an unwanted habit.

Step 3. Visualization. As you remain in a deeply receptive state, visualize the spirit realm with its myriad of colorful planes, each situated over the other like smooth layers of cirrus clouds stretched across the horizon. With your hands resting comfortably in your lap or to your sides and your palms turned upward, select a shimmering plane that stands out from the others and visualize a bright beam of light reaching from the plane to the palm of your hand. Think of your hands as your body's antennae to the universe as you sense the powerful infusion of the plane's energy, first in your hands and then throughout your body. Sense the attunement and balance that always accompany this experience. Once the infusion is complete, you can select other planes of color and interact with them one by one, depending on your preferences and needs. For goals related to health, fitness, and rejuvenation, interactions with iridescent planes of emerald are recommend. Planes of yellow are associated with enriched mental and social functions. Blue planes represent serenity, relaxation, and balance. For goals related to spirituality, interactions with planes of purple or indigo are recommended. An exceptionally radiant plane that commands your attention is typically appropriate for any pressing life situation.

Step 4. Affirmation. In your own words, affirm the empowering effects of your interactions with higher planes. Further affirm that the multiple higher planes of power are constantly available to you and receptive to your interaction with them.

Step 5. Post-script Cue. Affirm that you can at any moment activate the full empowering effects of this script by simply bringing your hands together to form the so-called *handclasp of power.* You can use that simple cue at will to generate an instant infusion of higher plane power related to the situation at hand.

Step 6. Exit and Conclusion. To end the script, give yourself permission to exit the trance or other receptive state. Take plenty of time to reflect on the experience and ways of using it to more fully empower your life. Journal your experience.

This script is one of the most effective self-empowerment programs known—its limits, if they exist at all, are unknown. It has been used with success to instantly break the smoking habit, generate highly creative ideas, accelerate learning, overcome persistent fear, lose weight, manage pain, retrieve past-life experiences, solve pressing problems, and even gain material wealth, to list only a few of the possibilities. Beginning now, you can use this script to empower your life as never before with enrichment, success, and happiness.

CONCLUSION

In this chapter, we have explored only a few scripts. We've found that each script has multiple applications and near-unlimited empowerment possibilities. They are flexible—you can easily adapt them to your present life situation. As noted, they are not limited to the trance state—they can be used during almost any responsive state, including the state of drowsiness preceding sleep.

Once mastered, the scripts presented in this chapter can become lifelong resources that increase in power with continued use. By making them a part of your everyday life, you have taken a major step toward the full realization of your potential for growth and greatness.

CHAPTER FIVE

PRACTICAL APPLICATIONS

We learn things, and then we have opportunities to apply what we know to new situations. Sometimes, simply because of its newness, we may think our new learning is too abstract or spiritual to have practical applications, or we may even think that a practical application for our new knowledge would somehow degrade it. Many times we don't even realize that our new learning can have practical applications.

Maybe we do learn new things for the pure enjoyment of learning, or the enjoyment of a new craft, or subject interests that are well outside those of our profession or career, and we assume there to be nothing practical involved. Yet, really, whatever we learn becomes part of our universal tool box and is applied to whatever we're working on, whether we realize it or not. Even the most seeming spiritual knowledge contributes to our well being, and that itself shows its practicality.

Yes, the date a particular European king ordered an obscure royal cousin beheaded may not itself provide for any application we can think of, but it still is background information about that historical period that may prove indirectly helpful when dealing with a client of the same national background. Practicality is not an isolated compartment with dedicated content.

Nevertheless, we undoubtedly do have more pertinent situations for our expertise, and the ability to remember more about a personal encounter could be helpful. Or, having more complete memories related to a particular situation would give us a more complete picture. Or, recalling a forgotten fact could shed new light on a current problem.

Or, more importantly, there is intelligence and wisdom locked up with those memories and having complete access to the subconscious mind will expand our conscious awareness and abilities. Just like your computer memory, your subconscious recorded the data but when it's not filed correctly, it becomes lost. You need to fix your filing system. You will learn several consciousness-expanding techniques in the next chapter, but here we will deal with one of the most powerful life-style changes you can make, and then add a few simple tricks that will be useful almost any time.

ACCESSING MEMORIES
IN THE SUBCONSCIOUS MIND

There are several ways to access those memories, but the most important step you can take is the *intention* to be organized. In the Introduction, we described several techniques and placed a lot of emphasis on the value of journaling. If you are now doing this, employing a good bookkeeping system on your computer, and are now filing both your computer data and paper materials, you are well on the way to organizing your subconscious mind even though you are not doing it consciously.

We will talk about it again and again. It being the *journal* We're going to provide a sample of a daily journal at the end of this book that you can copy on to your computer as a template if you'd like, or just use as an outline. We will give further emphasis to journaling in chapter six when we describe particular exercises for consciousness integration, but the value of a journal starts with the very first step.

The idea of keeping a journal should not be overwhelming. Yes, you already have a busy day but when you combine the journal with a dream diary and a scheduler plus a health record, you see the value increase as it is matched by the efficiency of a combined format. Of course, if you already use a scheduler on your computer, such as "Outlook," you will want to continue it, but the point remains that *an organized life is not only more efficient but far more productive.*

JOURNALING FOR LIFE

What is this amazing thing that happens when we put it down on paper? It doesn't really matter if you write with an old-fashioned quill pen in a lovely bound blank book of handmade paper or if you use your computer's word processor and never print it out. As long as you've recorded it, and it is saved so that you can review it at will, the physical act will have served to move your subjective experience from 'inside' to 'outside' where the conscious mind can interact with it. And, then, when you later read it and muse or meditate upon it, you take it back 'inside' for the subconscious mind to add to it with linked memories and fixtures of the astral, subconscious, world.

You are bringing 'inner' and 'outer' together into the richness of the Whole.

Compare that, for a moment, with the typical entry into your day planner or scheduling software. There, usually, you are only recording an appointment so that you will be reminded of it in time to do something. However, instead you could look ahead and see that you have a particular appointment that you need to prepare for, to think about in advance, perhaps even meditate about—calling upon your subconscious to add information and insight to the equation.

You are this time bringing 'outer' and 'inner' together with the additional power of the subconscious and perhaps the collective unconscious. You are acting as a whole person.

It is truly unfortunate that so few people actually work with their subconscious mind in such a directly beneficial manner. Self-empowerment comes from blending the conscious and subconscious minds together in beneficial interaction. To get the maximum benefit, we need to train and educate both while building bridges to engage each in our chosen projects.

Look at what happens with a trained tennis player: After learning and perfecting this kind of stroke and that kind of stroke, learning how to move with speed and sureness to and from the most challenging areas of the court, learning to return a high ball with power into the very edge of the opposite court, and so on—there's always more to learn. Those are the things that are learned in the outer world. In the meantime, in the inner world, the future champion is becoming able to intuitively anticipate the opponent's positions and moves, to intuitively know how to stroke the ball with a reverse spin, and to intuitively know when to deliver the *coup de grace.*

Inner and outer work together in perfect harmony and unity in the whole person. To put it bluntly: *Winners apply the training and skills of both subconscious and conscious minds focused together on a single project; Losers don't!* The self-empowered person is a winner, whether in the daily job, in the public arena, or in spiritual endeavor.

MEMORY TRICKS AND SELF-HYPNOSIS

Word association. This is one of the most familiar of the little tricks to recall specific memories from the subconscious. Simply make a list, or talk it over with someone, of words you feel have a connection with the forgotten name, word, fact, or event.

It may not work immediately, but having started the process it usually produces results. It's like having several fishing lines of different lengths in the water at the same time—eventually *your* fish will bite.

Sleep on it. This can be even more effective when dealing with a larger issue. Frame the memory you are looking for as a question, and sleep on it. Every evening, as you drop off to sleep, repeat the question until you get the answer you want.

Or, you may realize you haven't asked exactly the right question— so change it. If the missing information is important, it will eventually come to the surface.

Ask and it shall be given. Somewhat the same as the above, the point remains that you won't get the answer until you ask the question. The secret in all these memory tricks is intermittent persistence: ask the question, and give the subconscious time to come back with the answer. If it doesn't, repeat as necessary.

MULTIPLYING MIND POWER

Talk about it, ask about it. Putting two or more heads together is very productive. Now you are multiplying 'brain power,' although it really isn't brain power but that of your greater consciousness working through several people on the same project.

Obviously, this has more applications than just one person recalling where he left his car keys! *The Group Mind is like nuclear power.* The challenge is to keep your group organized and focused. There are different techniques for this, ranging from ritual to social. A ritual can be simple or complex—from simply starting a meeting with a prayer appealing to a 'higher power' or a concise statement of the problem and an outline of its importance to an elaborately staged drama. At the other extreme, a group that meets together in a shared goal—such as the finance committee of a local bank—can start with a simple lunch, and then focus on the work of the day for a specific time frame, perhaps of no more than thirty minutes.

What is always necessary with the Group Mind is leadership and focus. Do not deviate once you are focused on the problem: no references to weekend sports, political news, or even other problems. Set the rules for productivity, and adhere to them.

Now, look back over these memory tricks and see how they all actually involve some of the principles of self-hypnosis. Seeing that, you can now add the elements of self-hypnosis you've learned in this book to any of these techniques: Relaxation, Calmness, Goal Setting, and Focus. You don't need to wait for your regular times for self-hypnosis, meditation, or self-empowerment exercises. Your subconscious mind is always with you and always ready to help, but the channels of communication between conscious and subconscious have become cloudy so you have to work at it.

A self-empowered person knows that, and knows how to employ self-hypnosis in every situation.

HEALTH AND FITNESS

Better health and fitness through self-hypnosis is based on the simple premise that the potential for wellness exists in everyone. That potential, which is an inner healing force, is an integral part of your total being that's always receptive to your health and fitness needs. Through self-hypnosis, you can generate a powerful mind, body, and spirit interaction that unleashes an abundant flow of healthful energy and focuses it directly on specific health and fitness goals. Here are a few examples.

- You can become mentally, physically, and spiritually attuned and balanced, conditions that are conducive to better health and fitness.

- You can reduce negative stress and reverse its wear and tear effects.

- You can discover new ways of managing pain, to include reducing its intensity and redirecting it as healing energy.

- You can break unwanted habits that are detrimental to your health and fitness.

- You can discover higher sources of healing energy and master ways of interacting with them.

Programs designed to achieve each of these important goals using self-hypnosis are at last available to everyone. The effectiveness of each health and fitness program, like other applications, depends largely on clearly formulated goals, successful induction of the trance state, positive affirmations of success, relevant visualization, and in many instances, post-hypnotic suggestions for later use in activating or reinforcing the empowering effects of the trance experience. Upon exiting the trance state, taking a few moments to reflect on the experience and then journaling the experience can markedly increase its empowering effects. Through repeated practice, you can improve the effectiveness of each program.

In the discussion that follows, we'll examine several self-hypnosis programs related to specific health and fitness goals. Each program requires approximately thirty minutes in a comfortable setting free of distractions. The programs were developed in a laboratory setting and tested for effectiveness with volunteer subjects of wide-ranging characteristics, including extensive age differences.

MANAGING STRESS

Our studies of self-hypnosis often showed that the trance induction process alone can be empowering. For instance, deep relaxation when used to induce hypnosis is an excellent stress management exercise, independent of any subsequent application of the trance state. That being said, induction programs using progressive relaxation are among the most often preferred for health and fitness goals, including those that focus on prevention and pain management.

Interactive Relaxation is a self-hypnosis program that's appropriate for almost any health concern for which excessive stress is a contributing factor. It's based on the supremacy of the mind over the body and the capacity of the mind to directly influence physiology. While recognizing the potentially productive effects of positive stress that can be both motivating and energizing, this program equips you with the skills required to manage excessive or negative stress. With repeated practice, the program generates an empowered state that reduces negative stress and ameliorates its harmful wear and tear effects, including fatigue, increased susceptibility to illness, and sleep disturbances, to mention but a few. It recognizes the detrimental effects of stress on internal organs and the urgency of managing excessive stress that, in the long term, can be lethal. Fortifying your immune system, accelerating healing, managing pain, and preventing illness are each within the scope of this program. Before beginning the program, it's important to specify your goals in positive terms. Enter them in your journal and affirm your intent to achieve them. Here's the program.

Step 1. Induction. To induce the trance state, settle back and take in a few deep breaths, exhaling slowly. While resting comfortably, close your eyes and slowly relax your body from your forehead downward. Take plenty of time to sense relaxation soaking deeply into every muscle, fiber, and joint of your body. Upon becoming fully relaxed, let yourself enter the trance state by counting slowly backward from five to one while interspersing suggestions of going deeper and deeper into hypnosis. Upon the count of one, you can deepen the trance state if needed by visualizing a tranquil scene while again counting slowly backward from five to one.

Step 2. Stress Management. Focus your attention on the bright, peaceful center of your being. As you focus on that center deep within, let the brightness of that space slowly expand to infuse your total being—mind, body, and spirit—with the glow of serenity, self assurance, and peace. Affirm in your own words that you can at any moment infuse your total being with power to cope effectively with any situation at hand by simply focusing your attention on that quiet center of power within. You can at this point specify other goals and affirm your power to achieve them. Visualize yourself having achieved your goals while sensing the emotional satisfaction of your success.

Step 3. Conclusion. To end the trance state, simply count slowly from one to five with interspersed suggestions of being alert and fully awake. Record the experience in your journal and take a few moments to reflect on its empowering effects.

Interactive Relaxation is one of the best programs known for managing chronic pain and the stress associated with it. For that application, the program recognizes the complexity of pain and the importance of consulting with your physician in managing it. By focusing on the pain and then suggesting that the intensity of the pain is giving way to a dull, wooden feeling, you can often reduce the pain and tension resulting from it. You can then use visualization, both during hypnosis and afterward as a post-hypnotic cue, to bathe the area of pain with bright, healthful energy that not only reduces pain but promotes healing at the same time.

LOSING WEIGHT

For managing weight, self-hypnosis can strengthen motivation and ensure success not only in losing weight but keeping it off as well.

The New You is a program specifically designed to achieve that two-fold goal while promoting overall health and fitness. The program combines powerful affirmations along with imagery designed to give substance to your stated goal. Here's the program. Prior to induction, state your goal and enter it in your journal

1. **Induction.** Induce the trance state using either the interactive relaxation program as discussed above or the eye-fixation approach, in which attention is centered on a shiny object, such as a thumbtack situated on the wall or ceiling to facilitate a slightly upward gaze, as suggestions of relaxation and drowsiness are presented. Such deepening techniques as reverse counting and relaxing imagery can be used as needed to deepen the trance state.

2. **Application.** State your goal of weighing a certain amount, and then visualize yourself weighing that exact amount, perhaps while standing unclothed before a full length mirror. Let that visualized image of yourself become firmly engraved in your mind. Accompany the visualization with such affirmations as *this is the true me; I will succeed in achieving my goal of weighing exactly (state amount); day by day, I will follow a healthful diet; and I am now fully empowered to lose weight and keep it off.*

3. **Conclusion.** To exit hypnosis, count forward from one to five accompanied by suggestions of becoming fully awake and alert. Take a few moments to reflect on the experience and reaffirm your determination to achieve your goal. Journal the experience.

You can repeat this program as often as needed to strengthen your determination to lose weight and keep it off. You can use visualization of yourself having achieved your goal to instantly build your determination to succeed. Upon successfully achieving your goal, you can continue to use this program to ensure your continued success.

BREAKING THE SMOKING HABIT

Breaking the smoking habit through self-hypnosis is based on the premise that the need to stop smoking can overpower the need to smoke. To achieve that goal, a program called *New Beginning* is designed to build a powerful resolve to quit smoking accompanied by changes in the self-concept from being a smoker to a nonsmoker. It's an instant, all-or-nothing approach, sometimes called the *shotgun method*. While a residual need to smoke may in some cases remain, the program generates in an instant a new concept of you as a successful nonsmoker. Prior to induction, state your goal of being a nonsmoker and record it in your journal.

Here's the program, which requires approximately thirty minutes in a comfortable setting free of distraction.

1. **Induction.** While comfortably relaxed in a seated or reclining position, induce the trance state by spreading the fingers of either hand and then slowly relaxing them as you count backward from ten to one. Accompany your counting with interspersed suggestions of becoming more and more relaxed and going deeper and deeper into hypnosis. Upon the count of one, you can deepen the trance state as needed through visualization of a peaceful scene accompanied by additional reverse counting and suggestions of becoming more relaxed and going deeper.

2. **Stop Smoking Now.** Once in a successful trance state, affirm in your own words your decision to stop smoking along with such positive affirmations as: Beginning now, I am a nonsmoker. If I'm offered a cigarette, I'll respond, "*I am now a nonsmoker.*" If I find myself thinking of smoking, I'll remind myself, "*I am now a nonsmoker.*" When I observe others smoking, I'll remind myself, "*I am now a nonsmoker.*"

3. **Conclusion.** End the trance state by slowly counting from one to five with interspersed suggestions of becoming alert and fully awake. Journal the experience.

Although this program uses a single session to break the smoking habit, subsequent sessions can be used to reinforce the program's effectiveness by extinguishing any residual urge to smoke while building a powerful expectation of complete success. You can use the simple affirmation: *I am now a nonsmoker,* at any moment as a post-hypnotic empowerment cue to ensure your complete success in breaking the smoking habit.

BALANCE AND ATTUNEMENT

Perhaps nothing is more crucial to your overall health and fitness than a state of mental, physical, and spiritual attunement. This program, called *Power Beyond*, is based on the premise that abundant sources of healthful energy exist not only within your own being, but in dimensions beyond the self as well. Furthermore, those sources are constantly receptive to your interaction. Prior to inducing the trance state, state your goal and enter it in your journal. Here's the program.

1. **Induction.** Induce the trance state using the interactive relaxation program as previously presented.

2. **Attunement and Balance.** While in the deeply relaxed trance state, note the sense of complete inner peace. Affirm that all your cares are rolled away. Take time to experience that deep state of serenity and quietness within. Focus your attention on your solar plexus as the center of your being and visualize light radiating from it to infuse your full body with healthful, glowing energy. Visualize the light emanating from within reaching beyond you and stretching to infinity to unite with the highest sources of power. Note your sense of complete inner balance and full attunement with the universe. Allow that state to continue until it seems to have run its course, and then affirm: *I am now fully balanced and attuned to the powers within myself and beyond. Nothing is impossible for me in this state of complete oneness.* You can at this point visualize your body fully bathed in

bright, healthful energy. You can focus your attention on specific health needs, to include particular organs and their functions.

3. **Conclusion.** Conclude the program by counting slowly from one to five with interspersed suggestions of alertness and wakefulness. On the count of five, reflect on the experience and your sense of peaceful balance and attunement. Enter the experience in your journal.

You can dramatically increase this program's effectiveness through repeated practice, especially in the evening hours. It's an excellent program for promoting healthful sleep and dreaming.

Each health and fitness program presented here is flexible and can easily be personalized to fit your own interests and needs. Through repeated practice, you can dramatically improve your ability to enter the trance state and apply it to achieve even your most complex health and fitness goals. Reflecting on the trance experience and keeping a journal of your success can further advance the empowering effects of each program. You will soon discover that your use of self-hypnosis to promote health and fitness will become rapidly generalized to enrich and empower your total life.

SELF-PROGRAMMING FOR SUCCESS

"Success" is a very meaningful word and a powerful concept. There is no limit to the goals we can wrap into that one word. While "being successful" is commonly applied to the attainment of fame and fortune, and power, it also defines any and every accomplishment. Success is meeting your goals. Success is employing your talents and skills to bring an intended benefit. Success is living your life well. Success is the 'magic bullet' that protects you and by extension your loved ones. Success is happiness and fulfillment.

Success is also a mindset that attracts more success. *How do we get started?* We learn one simple rule: "Like attracts Like." We observe that money attracts money, that beauty attracts beauty, and that power attracts power. *What do you want?* Start with a little bit of it and more will be attracted to it.

All true, but *what's more powerful than money and beauty?* " in self." And more powerful than a little bit of money or beauty are the images you plant in the subconscious that will bring you the wealth and happiness and other things you desire when you employ the principles of self-empowerment and self-hypnosis we're teaching you in this book.

For the self-empowered person, success is a constant companion.

Step 1. Follow your preferred procedures of induction outlined earlier in Chapter Three.

Step 2. Identify your goal of success. *What does success mean to you? How does it relate to your sense of self, to your education and training, to your dreams of completeness and fulfillment, and so forth?*

The important difference here between specific goal identification and your goal of success is that Success is the Big Picture. It's not just becoming the President-Elect of the United States, but your vision of you as the historical figure of the President for the next four or eight years, and what you expect to accomplish and how you will be seen.

At the same time that this is your big picture of success, it doesn't mean that all else is excluded. Condoleezza Rice was not only Secretary of State but she was also a respected concert pianist. Hilary Clinton not only became Secretary of State but she remained a wife and a mother. The big picture is inclusive of your major success but also all other important parts of your life related to that success. Success is who you are in the outer world.

Step 3. Write it down. Always write your success picture down. Review it from time to time, change it as time goes by to reflect the changes in your life but still remembering the successful person you are. And as those changes occurred you may have a second successful career. After a successful career as a leading residential architect in San Francisco, you may retire and become a successful photographer of unique homes and publisher of photographic books. Your life can be fulfilled in more than one dimension.

Success is evolutionary because you are always evolving. You are never just one thing, but your big picture should represent the success of who you are now.

Step 4. Analyze the challenges. There is always a challenge, no matter who you are and where you are. Even at the peak of your success, there are challenges and your analysis of the Big Picture must recognize those challenges and how you will successfully meet them. It is not the details of how you as President will win the 'War on Terror,' but how you will see yourself as the President who successfully won the War on Terror.

Step 5. Write down your expectations. Always write it down. It is always essential to bring the inner vision into outer reality and the first step in this process is to write it down in your journal. And then to review your journal to bring that vision back inside to modify it as things progress, and then externalize the modified vision by writing it down too.

Step 6. Write the I AM sentence. When dealing with the Big Picture of your success, remember to keep it flexible and evolutionary. "I AM successfully fulfilling my job as a great defense attorney." It is important not to confuse the big picture with the many individual goals that will be part of your life every day. Your success as a great defense attorney is not a function of your weight loss program, which may be represented in the sentence "I AM slim." The big picture is more than the sum of those little pictures we discussed previously as goals.

Step 7. Memorize it.

Step 8. Visualize it. Close your eyes and visualize the sentence in White Letters against a black background. As you see it, speak the sentence with your inner voice.

Step 9. Image or Symbol. Now, silently ask your subconscious mind to produce a simple image or symbol to fully represent that sentence. This is the symbol of your success. This is your 'talisman' of success. It's like a very personal and very real 'Good Luck Charm.' Your subconscious mind has called out to the collective unconscious to find a powerful symbol of your success. Memorize it, and draw it—no matter what your artistic skills are.

Step 10. Memorize it. See your image or symbol in the same mental scene as your "I AM" sentence. Know that you now have the power to make your dream come true.

Step 11. The New Reality. Remember that you are leaving an old reality behind and replacing it with a new reality that is you as your successful self. See yourself in this new reality as if it has already happened. Make this your future NOW. Feel yourself in the new reality, repeat your vision of the image and your "I AM" sentence together, and hear your inner voice say it. Tie it all together so any time you repeat the sentence in your mind, you know that what is accomplished in the Inner World is manifesting in the physical world, and that your body, mind, and spirit are working together to bring this about.

You are a self-empowered person and success is your constant companion. Success is not just momentary, but it is you always meeting your individually stated goals. All those accomplished goals are like beads strung on a necklace that is as intrinsic to your self image as it is your 'badge of office.'

BUILDING SELF-CONFIDENCE

Self-confidence is *Belief in your Self.* Like success, it is with you all the time but it's easier to find books on self-confidence than on success. There are hundreds of them and there have been thousands of lectures on the subject. They're all good, but they lack one important recognition: *Self-confidence is empty until you know who your self is, and where it is that you are going.*

We've emphasized the importance of self-understanding elsewhere in this book, and in chapter seven we suggest the birth horoscope as one approach, but this is not a book on astrology or on self-understanding. At the same time, your vision of success is fundamental to your self-confidence because it is where you want to go. Your starting point is who you are and the ending point is where you're going. Confidence deals with what lies in between those two points.

Make a checklist to establish the knowledge and skills you need to become successful and another to represent the knowledge and skills you have now. Many of your goals will involve matching those two lists together. If your success vision requires knowledge and skill in the practice of law, and you do not currently have that, one of your intermediate goals must be to earn a degree and pass the bar exams. If your success vision requires the ability of an orator, then your intermediate goals should include the study of rhetoric and the practice of debate, and perhaps voice training, skills as an actor, and the study of posture, stance, and appearance.

Self-confidence involves recognizing those intermediate goals, establishing a plan with a schedule for their accomplishment, and believing in your ability and capacity to meet each of the individual challenges. Self-confidence is not over-confidence or empty-confidence; it is an attitude built on realistic plans and expectations.

Yes, your attitude of confidence includes satisfaction with your appearance, your social skills, and your self-representation. It is built on realism and the ability to see yourself as you are and as how you want to be, and knowing that you can bridge the gap between the two. It is composed of energy, awareness, and determination. It is powered by ambition.

Your procedure is to bring all these things together and condense them into a single I AM sentence and vision just as we previously outlined, and when in trance, express and see yourself accordingly. See an image of yourself walking, smiling, standing, and gesturing with self-confidence, and know that it is you.

CHANGING YOUR APPEARANCE

Changing your appearance is a realistic goal no matter what the circumstance. It should be part of your vision of success and your expression of self-confidence, and it starts with an assessment of who you are, your appearance now, and the appearance you want, with a realistic perspective on the road in between.

Women, for the most part, have an advantage over men in this regard because they have been dressed by adults, their hair brushed, and they've been taught how to make themselves attractive, and praised with each success, etc. And there is a vast industry of clothing, cosmetics, beauticians, magazines, advice programs, exercise programs, counselors, and peer support to address their needs. They have learned to 'dress for the occasion.' They have not been limited to appearing for one role only.

But men and women both may have personal challenges of weight, posture, attitude, and unrealistic expectations. It is unrealistic to think you can become six foot four in height if you are only five foot three now. On the other hand, nearly anyone with hair can become a blond if that is their wish. If your attitude is that appearance shouldn't matter, then there is no likelihood that you can change until you decide you want to.

As in every program, the first step is to assess where you are now and where you want to go, and then to recognize the steps in between. Those steps can become goals to be met in the process of self-hypnosis we've already discussed. But there is one other, bigger step that can be taken using self-hypnosis: you can develop the image you desire and imprint it in your subconscious so that all the steps you take are guided by that self-image. You can see it as the process of *sculpting* body, face, hair, clothing, posture, etc. to match the imprinted self-image.

It's a very personal process, and a very meaningful one, because appearance is not as superficial as it seems. The appearance that includes glowing health is very powerful in guiding the body in that direction. The appearance of professional competency is likewise very powerful in guiding the person to fulfill the image. The body and the expressive personality are quite plastic and can be molded to meet the self-image you establish. Even the appearance of great wealth can attract wealth—but with many reservations about ethics, legalities, and practicalities.

Programming the image you desire is based on the principles already outlined for you. Essentially, you describe the image you desire, picture it, write your I AM sentence, and develop a symbol to represent it. You embed that sentence and symbol 'loaded' with the description and actual image in the subconscious. They then inspire the subconscious mind to bring this image into reality.

ATTRACTING WEALTH

In recent years, the power of attraction, particularly in relation to wealth, has been very much in the public eye. Authors of books on the subject have appeared on all the major talk shows, reviews and articles have been in print media and all over the Internet, the subject has been sermonized (positively) in the mega churches, numerous experts have positioned themselves as consultants and counselors, and the *Grande Dame* of mass marketing, Oprah Winfrey, has said she's used it all her life.

The power of attraction has a rich literary heritage going back to *The Power of Positive Thinking* by Norman Vincent Peale, *Think and Grow Rich* by Napoleon Hill, *The Science of Getting Rich* by Wallace Wattles, *As a Man Thinketh* by James Allen, and many more titles. And the power of attraction is by no means limited to attracting wealth, nor is wealth defined purely by money.

MONEY, MONEY, WHO'S GOT THE MONEY?

Money isn't what it used to be. Unfortunately, money is not easily understood and it's not easily talked about because of the emotional attachments involved. Money involves security, it buys food and shelter, it's an investment set aside for retirement, it's a resource enabling people to gain an education of choice and thus opening up jobs that are enjoyable and fulfilling, it represents and is power, and many more things.

Only a few hundred years ago, money was just "hard currency." It came mostly in the form of gold or silver coins and the way one accumulated more money essentially meant someone else had less money. Wealth could consist of gold and silver coins as well as jewels, land, castles, and slaves. Even people who didn't think of themselves as slaves were dependent on the landowner, the local ruler, the man who controlled an army, and the Church that controlled the hereafter.

You couldn't really *attract* this kind of wealth, and it was very difficult to earn much of it. You could steal it, just as the local ruler could send his army to steal land and property from some other ruler.

With that kind of wealth there were no public hospitals, schools, or welfare programs.

Then there came money lending and a new kind of currency was born that involved paper, trust, and eventually laws governing property and the enforcement of contracts. This new kind of money involved money itself earning money in the form of interest and later in the form of shares in the gains resulting from financing ventures such as wars, piracy, mining, and the cultivation of land to produce surplus crops of food and fiber.

With the coming of surplus, some wealth would be turned back into hard assets, often in the form of jewelry, and in some cultures gold and silver jewelry would be soldered on to women's wrists and ankles to secure household wealth, and to display it. Later, surplus was invested in larger homes and richer furnishings both for home and women's bodies. For many women, attracting wealth became a matter of more jewelry.

Money lending turned into banking and banking turned into finance. People lent their savings to the banker in exchange for modest interest, and the banker in turn lent it out—leveraged several times—to finance more ventures. At a certain point in modern history, technology replaced slave labor with wages and wage earners could use their savings for education and for investments to improve their lot.

With each progressive stage, money became less "hard" and wealth more 'occult' based on paper based on other paper and trust based on other trust. Such wealth can move freely about and can be 'attracted' because it is no longer tied to hard assets. No longer based on hard assets, wealth can easily diminish in fluctuating exchange values and even disappear because of irresponsible behavior of trusted financial people and government regulators.

What Real Wealth Is

Before we can attract wealth, we have to understand what it really is. Real Wealth, today, is the capacity to create wealth. Investment capital flows to the person who can increase its value significantly. Yes, some wealth is still gifted to beautiful women, but fewer women today think that "Diamonds are a girl's best friend." Wealth, particularly in the form of hard assets, can be stolen, and wealth in any form can be diminished and lost through abuse, fraud, manipulation, bad management, ignorance, and greed.

In contemporary society, men and women both see work and creativity as the source of both income and wealth. Education and training prepare a person to earn income, and quality performance leads to increased income. Surplus can be invested in various assets and set aside in programs for retirement and recreation, funding of college education for the children, and in further education and training for self-improvement.

What do we really mean when we talk of "attracting wealth"?

THE LAND OF OPPORTUNITY

Just as America was early on seen as the "land of opportunity," so today there remain many opportunities to create wealth.

What we really mean when speaking of attracting wealth is to attract the opportunities to create wealth. Such opportunities come in many forms:

1. Those for more education and training. Good performance in school and on the job can attract scholarships and training programs, advancing earning potential.

2. Sometimes it's who you know. Building relationships can open many opportunities in sales and marketing, opening the way for higher performance; in connecting with people who will recognize skills and creativity who in turn can open doors for you to produce at a higher level; and in recognizing talent in performance arts and bridging the way to appropriate development.

3. Connecting to capital for investment in new innovations and enabling sound management for their development.

4. The Right Time and Place. Sometimes it appears like 'pure luck' that you're the one who can provide what is needed to someone else. Being there may be a function of intuition, or of awareness, of activities in the field and area of interest.

5. Lightning Strikes. The idea 'out of the blue' that becomes a new success story.

How Do You Attract These and Other Opportunities?

- By knowing your capabilities, and thinking along creative lines for the opportunities that would benefit from them.

- By believing in yourself and having confidence that your capabilities will be recognized.

- By being an "attractor." Visualize yourself as a magnet attracting opportunities to yourself. You can use self-hypnosis to plant this vision in your subconscious.

- To whatever extent possible, use the "Like attracts Like" principle by surrounding yourself with the accessories of the talents, skills, etc. that represent your dreams. This does not mean spending money to look wealthy, but it does mean reading the trade and professional publications related to your goals, joining professional and trade organizations, attending conferences and conventions, etc.

- If your dream involves the performing arts or particular trades, to whatever extent that is appropriate and practical, dress the part. That doesn't mean wearing a welder's garb when you are at church, but it may mean wearing a simple emblem or talisman that symbolizes welding to you.

There it is. The "magic is in the believing and in creating the field of opportunities." Do all the right things, as described, and believe in your heart and soul that what you dream will come to pass.

THE GROUP MIND

"Group Mind"—*what does that phrase suggest to you?* Probably it reminds you of other phrases like Brain Trust, Brainstorming, and Brain-Busting.

Back in the early 1930s, there was a group of high-level academics who helped then President-Elect Franklin Delano Roosevelt formulate what became known as the "New Deal" to meet the economic crisis of the Great Depression. They were known as FDR's "Brain Trust." Similar groups have been assembled in similar circumstances to help other short-term planning in government and nongovernment situations. But, that's not what we mean by a *Group Mind*.

Commonly, groups and teams of people will get together for "Brainstorming" sessions around a central theme or problem. People will rapidly call out spontaneous ideas for further exploration, and after the initial list is quickly reduced to a few of the most interesting, these will be further discussed. But, that's not what we mean by a *Group Mind*.

Something similar has been adapted around "brain-busting" and "mind-busting" in the form of intelligent games of adults and kids. But, again, that's not what we mean by a *Group Mind*.

Both Brain Trust and Brainstorm touch upon the idea of Group Mind as they bring people together to work on a common objective. When these groups work well, there comes a feeling that the members are parts one of another and a sensation of being united in something *above* them. Sometimes there will seem to be psychic phenomena at work when two or more people will shout out the same word or idea together or simultaneously leap to their feet in enthusiasm.

Now, let's try to do this deliberately and continuously for a group of people regularly meeting—or *not even having to meet together physically.*

The Group Mind in the Kitchen Cabinet

The phrase "kitchen cabinet" was applied to the small, unofficial group of advisors of U.S. President Andrew Jackson, who had more influence than did his official cabinet of government officers who, like department managers in a business, are more often concerned with their own fields of responsibility than they are with the whole enterprise.

The Kitchen Cabinet worked more like several minds all functioning through a single person. It wasn't as if all the members of the group were each advising the President on his agenda, but more that there was a single mind elevated above the entire group that was doing the thinking. We see the same phenomenon when a flight of birds or a school of fish seems to change direction instantly as a single unit.

Thus a Group Mind is truly mind power multiplied many times and raised to a higher power, and the image of it floating in space above the group is imaginatively realistic. Imagine for yourself how it would be to have the collective power of even just two or three other minds united together and focused on the resolution of a single problem.

Think carefully about this, for it is *not* the same as having two or three other people offering you their advice and expertise; rather, it is more like having one person with all the expertise, all the experience, all the creative and intuitive ability, and all the psychic power plus the ability to reach into the collective unconscious of these many people all in one single mind. It's more than just having two or three or how ever many times the brain power, for it's that much greater psychic power calling up power from the collective unconscious and hence drawing upon the knowledge and experience of all who have gone before to focus on the one problem or challenge that you place on the group agenda.

Building the Group Mind

How can we create a Group Mind? Sometimes this happens more or less spontaneously, as when the Catholic Cardinals come together to kiss the ring of the new Pope, and oftentimes it does happen in a sporting event or political rally—sometimes with terrible results if something triggers an angry crowd to mass action. But notice this: it rarely happens 'under orders' from the top down. You may have mass action as obedience to a command from the top, and you may get the potentially terrible consequences of mass emotional movement, but these do not give you the unity of emotion with thought and spirit that comes through a real Group Mind. Try to think these differences through to better understand how this amazing psychic 'technology' works.

Sometimes it happens automatically when members of a team or group come together in common purpose with shared enthusiasm for their work. Napoleon Hill, author of *Think and Grow Rich*, believed that this kind of Group Mind contributed to the fabulous business success of Andrew Carnegie, John D. Rockefeller, and others. We can add to that list more contemporary successes in business and science, but we have a further observation to make that groups working together seem to build psychic connections leading to shared behavior, shared thoughts, and even shared timing of physiological processes.

Mind Melding and the Reality of the Group Mind

It stands to reason that it is the psychic factor that is at the foundation of building a Group Mind. Through mental telepathy, minds can be "melded" together and hence function with multiplied power.

So, there we have it—the reality of the Group Mind coming about through working together in common purpose, with mutual respect, shared enthusiasm, and psychic melding. By understanding the process as it naturally occurs, we can deliberately create the Group Mind when opportunity and need is present.

To avoid confusion, we need to mention that while a Group Mind is common to volunteer organizations, and religious and magical groups, that is a phenomenon with many practical differences from the intentional Group Mind we're going to develop that we need not to go into here.

We need also to note one other important example of a spontaneous Group Mind, and that is the one that builds around the intimate couple's relationship to become a family Group Mind. That can become a very powerful psychic entity functioning to guard the household, opening the spiritual potentials of husband and wife, welcoming and promoting the growth and development of children, working to protect and extend the family's wealth, acting to benefit the family member's careers and their health, and so on.

With all the potential benefit you can see possible with these examples of the spontaneous Group Mind at work, think now of what can happen with intentionally constructed Group Minds! Speculate on what involvement the traditional wedding ceremony may have in forming the scaffold, so to speak, for that Family Group Mind; think how joint actions in buying a home or renting an apartment will act upon the structure; and consider the powerful charge of sexual energy in constantly melding body, mind, and spirit.

We are not going into the dynamics of the intentional construction and melding of the intimate couple's Group Mind in this book, but including mention of it here will give you much room for thought.

Our intention is to create a kind of 'super ego' that can endure as a group identity and function as an independent entity, just as a legal charter does for a corporation or partnership. That identity is more than a composite of its founders and current officers. When the documents are filed, the corporation can even have a horoscope and history that will show that its identity is very real.

To distinguish the intentional Group Mind constructed with the aid of self-hypnosis we are giving it a name: *The Empowered Group Mind.*

Constructing the Empowered Group Mind

The Empowered Group Mind is intended to bring to the group the multiplied power of those associated with the group both at any time for an individual to draw upon, and at other times when the entire group or most of them coordinate their times to focus on a common effort, either in a meeting at a physical location or at a distance through the established psychic connections.

We start with the individuals each (1) identifying the unifying common purpose, i.e., goal of their union, (2) giving their trust and respect to each other, (3) building enthusiasm by visualizing an image of their unity as accomplished, (4) dedicating the development and activation of their own psychic powers and the resultant benefits to the most people possible, and (5) establishing the rules for individual and group action.

Next, we have to manage the group itself, most often as called together by a leader, although it is important to note that because of the psychic element it is not actually necessary to meet or work together in a shared physical location. And then the leader, or members alternating in that role, must guide the process—whether discussion, research, brainstorming, scheduling, coordinating, or visualizing the completed project. Finally, the psychic element: all the participants need to consciously imagine the progress on the work and feel the excitement of its coming fruition.

Self-Hypnosis and the Empowered Group Mind

We've described the nature of the Group Mind and hinted at the practical benefits that may be achieved through its multiplied 'brain power,' but we can go much further through the practical application of self-hypnosis to this remarkable melding phenomenon.

You, and each of the other members individually, will want to follow your usual procedures of relaxation induction preparation. However, when it comes to identifying the goal for your self-hypnosis session, be sure to establish it as the building of a Group Mind involving yourself and the others making up what will be the initial group. Give a simple but meaningful name to the group and write down the names of the members. And develop a very simple but unique image to represent the group.* Obviously, all the members have to use the same name and image.

Develop a statement such as: "I AM part of the (name) Group Mind," and see its unique image floating in space above the heads of your group. Develop a second statement establishing the basic mission of the group: "The mission of (name) is (word or short phrase)." Keep it concise and comprehensive rather than limiting.

When doing your self-hypnosis for a specific goal shared by all the group members, agree on a simple sentence such as: "The Newport Group is focused on healing Brother Carl's shoulder." Ideally, with such an intention, you will all have a mental image of Brother Carl with his healed shoulder, but at the same time be picturing healing energy flowing toward and into the shoulder. You are imaging both the process and the accomplishment in one picture.

---

* One approach to a unique image is to make a sigil out of the group name: simply spell out the name in upper-case letters, eliminate any duplicates, and consolidate any lines so that you end up one single image.with

While the members can work together joined only by their psychic links, there is substantial benefit to having them physically together in their initial operations. A common procedure for that is standing in a circle with hands joined together or arms upon shoulders. Once the leader establishes the goal of their work along with an image of its accomplishment, a concise statement is chanted in unison: "Brother Carl's shoulder is healed." As the chant is repeated a little faster and louder with each time and healing energy is felt to circle around and around until the leader brings it to a climax with everyone shouting the phrase.

Such a healing operation is a good demonstration, and a good way to establish the unity of the group. It is important, however, to quickly move on to other projects and to practice working together joined only psychically. Each group will have to develop their own procedure for this, usually picturing themselves as they were when last physically together.

It is also important for each to record the operation and their experience of it in their own journals and to share this with the other members, and to record the results when known.

One of your authors participated in such a group action, visualizing the distant recipient of the healing surrounded by healing light and energy and bringing it to a close with the shout, "She is healed." The recipient had no knowledge of the action, but she recorded that she was suddenly surrounded by light, felt the tumor in her throat grow hot, then cold, and then . . . *nothing!* She duly reported in to the clinic where the tumor was scheduled for removal, and *there was no tumor!*

Mutual Hypnosis

While the emphasis in this book is upon self-empowerment through self-hypnosis, it is worth mentioning the value of mutual hypnosis in establishing rapport among the group members. The practice of hetero-hypnosis is the same as self-hypnosis, but one person functions as the hypnotist and the other (or even several) as the subjects. In mutual hypnosis, after a level of trance is reached, the roles are reversed and the trance deepened. This can be repeated, alternating, several times, with the stated intention of strengthening the Group Mind in which they participate.

Included among the benefits of mutual self-hypnosis is the deepening of trust and respect among the members, and the increased strength of the group mind.

Group Practices to Build a Group Mind to Help in Team Projects

In the case of Teams established for short-term projects, some of the techniques and concepts mentioned previously apply more for the more permanent group that we can call a "committee" rather than a "team." Nevertheless there is a fundamental rule that applies to any number of people coming together:

When we listen to one another, we must commit to hear one another!

Even though the words above *listen* and *hear* are redundant, the truth in actual practice is that we often don't hear. We can debate which of the two words is active and which is passive, but the point remains that real listening or real hearing means understanding what the other person is saying. For our own purposes, we could say that "hearing is conscious listening." Such hearing is like concentrating on what is being said and understanding what is said to the extent that you forget even who is speaking. You hear only the idea.

A corollary rule for the functioning of our group, whether team or committee, is that *whoever is talking must speak to the entire group*, not just another person or two. The point is that each person must function as part of the group as a whole at all times. Even though the group only meets occasionally, the empowered group mind must be seen to exist all the time—not just when the people come together physically. And, yes, one person can be part of more than one empowered group mind so long as he or she keeps them separate.

And an important point to remember is that *once connected, we're always connected*, no matter how far apart we may be. That's one of the recognitions of quantum theory. Of course, we also know that the reality of togetherness diminishes with inactivity, and in the case of teams and committees the formal cessation of their activity does bring that togetherness to a 'near' zero.

As with an empowered group mind, it is vital to have leadership, agendas, and rules of conduct. At the same time, the more firmly established the group is, the less will these things obtrude. The most distinct difference between a team and a board or committee is that the team has a specific project, and a committee has an area of responsibility. In contrast, in business a department has a distinct function such as sales or customer service and a board is the group mind for the company as a whole.

Visualization of Steps Toward a Goal

Just as individuals must state goals and recognize the steps for their accomplishment, so must our team, committee, department, or board formally establish goals and analyze the steps necessary for their accomplishment. We should think of these as the 'permanent' agenda of the group. The effective group mind is as much a single entity as a single person with body, mind, and soul.

What gives the group meaning are the statement of goals and the development of the steps seen as necessary towards its accomplishment. These, along with the name and the list of members, must make up the items on the first agenda for the group. This starts the process of group mind empowerment. Once those steps are stated, the group members should visualize them each in their own way to mobilize the powers of their subconscious minds to the accomplishment of the set goal.

The empowered group mind is the most powerful engine of practicality we have.

See Appendix A for a sample of a suggested self-empowerment journal and magical diary.

CHAPTER SIX

INTERACTIONS BETWEEN "IN HERE" AND "OUT THERE"

There are two worlds—one is 'out there' (the world of our objective experience) and the other is 'in here' (the world of our subjective experience), and both are where we are. One appears to be *hard*, and the other *soft*, but where we are it's *just right*.

We think each is distinct from the other, but we should remember that both, just as does everything else, arise from the same primal source, the same Primal Universal Field. Two things with common origin are forever bound together, meaning there is unity behind the *appearance* of duality. Inner and outer are just two sides of the same thing and their unity is the third part of a trinity.

We know there is unity, but we also know there is duality—both perspectives are real and we can create an image of man with a dual vision looking within and looking without. Both visions are equally important but it is also important to remember their actual unity and to realize that we, as the Trinitarian factor, are the agent of that unity.

Remember the story of the natives unable to see the Spanish sailing ships because they had no previous experience with giant sailing ships at sea capable of carrying many men, horses, and weapons? There are several important lessons for us in that story:

1. Apparent empty space may not be empty at all.

2. A change of expectations can change our actual experience of the outer world.

    a. As subsets of the above, the mind can be trained to see things once invisible.

    b. The once invisible can become just as 'real' as that which was already visible.

    c. The once invisible is not necessarily dangerous or un-friendly—but can become so depending upon our future actions and reactions.

3. Outer and Inner are related through Consciousness.

4. In our study of inner and outer worlds, we need to use a single system that recognizes the commonalities between the two be-cause it is those commonalities that give us the means to con-trol the relationship between the two.

5. One characteristic of the conscious mind is to divide and label both the seen and the unseen as we attempt to grasp and un-derstand both internal and external phenomena.

It's this last point in particular that we want to discuss. Just be-cause we have mentally divided inner and outer worlds into various parts and given them names, it is important to remember that these are "man made" divisions and mostly not hard and fast partitions.

Where, for example, does the conscious mind end and subcon-scious mind begin? We speak as if there is a distinct boundary, like a 'fire wall' between conscious and unconscious, but of course there is not. Such distinctions are a convenience. They are real, yet what was in objective consciousness yesterday may be in the subconscious today, and be back in the conscious mind tomorrow. There are no hard and fast lines between objective and subjective, and yet each is distinct . . . for the moment.

The same is true of the distinctions between the physical plane and the astral plane. These planes are not layers like the lines of sediment on a canyon wall, yet that concept makes a good simile for some clairvoy-ants have described astral 'matter' as being of a *higher* vibration than physical matter. When discussing the astral body part of our Whole Being, we sometimes refer to it as the emotional body, or the subtle body, or the light body. We call it a 'body,' but there is no astral 'skin' defining and limiting it as there is skin for the physical body.

The point in this discussion is that there are no hard barriers to be overcome between physical and astral, or between the conscious mind and the subconscious. You don't need a 'passport' to move between these worlds, just as there is no wall between your physiological actions and your emotional reactions. Not only is there no barrier between the physical and astral worlds, but interactions are occurring all the time.

Our immediate goal is to integrate more of the subconscious with the conscious, and thus extend our awareness further into the astral world so that we function as more of a whole person. There are two things we want to do:

1. Better organize our life experiences and knowledge for greater and richer conscious accessibility;

2. Extend our capacity for 'the Whole View' so we more readily perceive at the astral level.

It is important for you to claim your 'wholeness.' *Why function as only part of the person you really are?* We are all here to learn and grow, but we are badly handicapped if we have an unorganized lifestyle, with inattention to details, and lack of comprehension relating to our general observations. Unfortunately, this failure applies to nearly everyone for the simple reason they lack appropriate training and our education was not inclusive of this at the youthful age when it would be formative. You've been *blind-sided* by an inadequate system that can be improved only as more educators themselves become Whole Persons.

Yes, you can do something about it. Systematic organization of your conscious experiences will carry over into an organization of your subconsciousness. The modern application of filing systems and scheduling of daily appointments begins a similar process for your subconscious mind, as do home bookkeeping and inventory systems. Even forgotten memories fall into an association with similar memories so that the recall of one will bring others with it.

Too often, people assume that when they choose to adopt a more 'spiritual life style,' everything will simply fall into place, that they will be surrounded with white protective light, and that angels will guide them through all difficulties. The truth is that life itself requires work, and through work we grow and learn. A more spiritual life-style requires additional spiritual work. Basic spiritual work is really the same as ordinary work—organized habits, respect for the process, planning, etc. In addition, a spiritual lifestyle calls for self-knowledge and self-understanding, meditation, training the image-making facility (i.e., disciplined imagination), daily reviews, etc., and *journaling*.

Journaling, in which you organize your experiences and observations into "systems," helps in both conscious and subconscious worlds where retrieval of a conscious memory will extend into the subconscious. Even nonphysical journaling is helpful; it's that recognition of 'this is like that' or 'not this, not that.' Nevertheless, the physical act of recording and filing completes the mental work of observation, analysis and recognition of details, comparison with other apparently similar things recalled as memories, and noting the meaning in relation to our goals. Journaling may sound challenging, but it really doesn't require more than a few minutes daily, and the real and subtle benefits are enormous and lifelong. The sooner you start, the easier it becomes and the faster the rewards will pile up.

The process starts with a system of observation and comparison, going beyond a mere diary of events. We will discuss a proven system for this later in this chapter.

There are ways to build connections and relationships even among your early experiences lost deep in the subconscious. And there are aids to help you awaken your dormant faculties. We can't instruct you fully in these systems and techniques here, but we will introduce you to them and guide you to some practical resources. It's worth remembering that through self-empowerment you are becoming a greater person, activating more of that ninety percent unused capacity.

THE ASTRAL WORLD AND
YOUR SUBCONSCIOUSNESS

It is difficult to clearly understand the astral world because it does not have the same kind of objective reality that the physical world does. Yet it exists and is real—but it's a different kind of reality while also being part of a shared reality with the physical world. It's another dimension, or 'phase,' but it's not separate from the physical world; it penetrates the physical world and is within it—sort of like a color that is mixed with others to produce something new.

We experience that astral world all the time, yet we have to understand things about it. There are three aspects to this that must be recognized to begin our discussion:

1. The astral world is where all your memories are recorded, and hence it is your subconscious. The astral light is responsive to feeling and thought impressions and records them just as your computer memory records your e-mails.

2. The Astral World is *formative* to the physical. Things exist on the astral prior to their manifestation in the physical. Your astral body acts as a *matrix* to the physical body. Your astral body is real but you can't feel it and most people can't see it.

3. The astral world is the *action domain* for the Imagination, for Emotion, Feeling, and Fantasy, and it is part of the total field of consciousness. The astral world is real, but its 'substance' is not only of a *higher vibration* but of a different kind of vibration than what we perceive in the physical world. And like physical matter, this substance is also energy. It has various names: *the Astral Light, Anima Mundi, Akasha, Aether, Chi, Prana, Spirit,* and others—all meaning the same thing but with a different perspective. You are actually creating in the astral world all the time.

We must remember that everything in the world originated and still originates from the primal universal field of consciousness that exists everywhere. It is not like a store or factory, but we might compare it to being able to go online and find a source for anything you can imagine. Once you specify what you want, it exists in the astral and, as you further define your specifications, it begins to manifest in the physical. Remember: *the astral is formative to the physical.*

QABALAH, CABBALA, AND KABBALAH

Include in this group QBL, the Hebrew word for "an oral tradition" referring to the esoteric system originally based on the mystical teachings of certain ancient Jewish rabbis and mystics. The various spellings you encounter represent different approaches to certain of the practices over the centuries among Christian mystics, Occultists, and traditional Jewish scholars. There are some other variations, thoughtfully justified by their advocates, which we will not develop here. And to make it plain and simple we will just accept the most common spelling, Kabbalah.

The Kabbalah provides us with the most complete and practical system for organizing and comparing our observations and experiences of both the objective and the subjective worlds. It is an ideal system to use with your journaling. We can't teach it all to you here, but will outline it sufficiently and recommend a few very valuable books for further study. While it is identified as 'Jewish Mysticism,' it has become something inclusive of mystical and magical practices, but even more an encyclopedia of 'correspondences' relating things and energies by their universal attributes and our experiences (called paths) of them joined in particular patterns on the Tree of Life, itself a comprehensive organizing principle.

The Kabbalah is a trustworthy guide, leading to a comprehension both of the universe and one's own self. The tree of life … is at once a symbolic map of the universe in its major aspects, and also of its smaller counterpart, man.

A Garden of Pomegranates, *xviii*

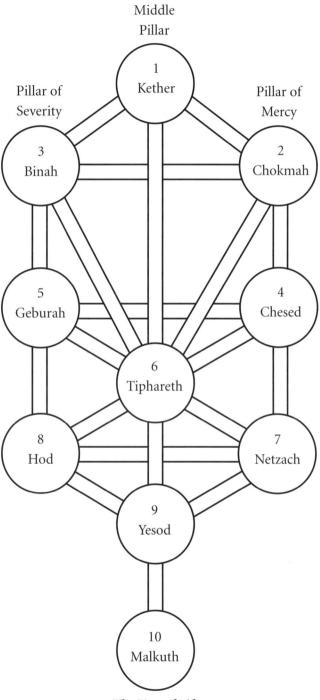

The Tree of Life

INNER AND OUTER—ONE MAP

The Kabbalah is a symbolic explanation for the origin of the Universe and Humanity, their relationship to the Creative Forces, and a systematic organization of existing knowledge and new experience. Its main 'construct' is the 'Tree of Life,' a schematic drawing organizing the relationships between ten spheres called "sephiroth" (the plural of "sephirah") connected by twenty-two Paths. The Tree of Life is a metaphor for the Body of God, and for men and women created in his image, for the Universe as all that is and for Man who lives within.

The sephiroth are aligned in three columns and are grouped variously into three triangles of three sephiroth each, leaving one lone sephirah at the bottom, or one triangle and a group of seven, or one triangle and a group of five and a group of two at the bottom, or two triangles and a group of four, and so on. The two side columns each have three sephiroth while the middle one has four. Each pattern brings the sephiroth into different energetic relationships stimulating different interactions. Other variations are also used. In addition, there is an eleventh sephirah that is 'hidden' and used in another manner. And there are three 'veils of negative existence' that precede the top sephirah.

The twenty-two Paths connecting the sephiroth are assigned to the twenty-two letters of the Hebrew alphabet and to the twenty-two Major Arcana of the Tarot. In another conception, there are four trees representing the four worlds—of the Archetypes, of Creation, Formation, and Action. The first ten numbered cards of each of the four suits of the Minor Arcana of the Tarot are assigned to the ten sephiroth, while the four 'Court Cards' of each suit are assigned to the four worlds represented as Trees of Life.

All the various ways of viewing the Tree as a whole, in parts, in different divisions, as four Trees together, viewed as from the front and then in reverse from the back, as placed on the human body, as seen in different perspectives from above and from below, in different color systems, etc. are ways to apply a universal formula both to Man and to the Universe to bring understanding to the various relationships physically, psychologically, magically and spiritually. Too, the four worlds of the Tree relate to the four primary bodies of Man: Physical, Astral, Mental, and Spiritual.

We say that everything is connected to something else, that each thing relates to other things, and that we are all one in spirit. The Kabbalah is the science of those connections and relationships, of the correspondences that allow substitution of one thing for another or the support of one thing by another, and of that which unifies all.

The Qabalistic alphabet is… an elaborate system of attributions and correspondences; a convenient method of classi|-fication enabling the philosopher to docket his experiences and ideas as he obtains them.

As experience increased, each letter and number would receive fresh accessions of meaning and significance, and by adopting this orderly arrangement, we would be able to grasp our inner life much more comprehensively than might otherwise be the case (enabling) . . . the student to do three main things: First, analyze every idea in terms of the Tree of Life. Second, to trace a necessary connection and relation between every and any class of idea by referring them to this standard of comparison. Third, to translate any unknown system of symbolism into terms of any known one by its means . . . bringing home to us the common nature of certain things, the essential difference between others, and the inevitable connection of all things. (A Garden of Pomegranates, *31–32*)

The Tree of Life is also used as a map that organizes the contents of the subconscious mind and opens doorways to the super conscious Mind and the collective unconscious. It's a treasure map to the riches of Spirit and sometimes to those of the practical world as well. It is also the foundation of magic, focusing the knowledge of mind and the energies of body and soul to control the physical manifestation of astral desire. *Nothing great in the world has ever been accomplished without passion* (George Wilhelm Friedrich Hegel, philosopher).

> *The Kabbalah reveals the nature of certain physical and psychological phenomena. Once these are apprehended, understood and correlated, the student can use the principles of magick to exercise control over life's conditions and circumstances not otherwise possible. In short, magick provides the practical application of the theories supplied by the Kabbalah.*
>
> (A Garden of Pomegranates, *xix*)

We will return to the Kabbalah later in this chapter. But there is one final quotation to consider at this point:

> *The Universe began not with an atom or a subatomic particle, but with a thought in the mind of God. This thought of Creation encompassed a world in which every human being would enjoy happiness and fulfillment, free from any form of chaos or pain. This is what the Creator desires and intends.*
>
> *But bringing about the realization of the Creator's desire is up to us. For the manifestation of complex fulfillment to take place, we need to evolve into our truest, greatest selves. In our thoughts, our feelings, and our actions, we need to erase negativity and replace darkness with Light. It is for this purpose that the teachings and tools of Kabbalah were given to all humanity.*
>
> (*By Rav Berg in the Introduction*, The Sacred Zohar)

TAROT—FROM INNER TO OUTER

The Tarot is familiar to us as 78 interesting picture cards most often seen as an entertaining practice of "fortune telling" and rumored to have its origin with the European Gypsies who received it from India, or was it ancient Egypt, or as invented to amuse certain rich noble families of Italy. In other words, no one knows for sure and each myth has its own meaning and adds another dimension to the system.

Perhaps it lacks ancient history and like the Kabbalah gained its present depth of esoteric and psychological power in a purely evolutionary manner that was formalized by certain occultists adapting it via the Kabbalah to a method not of fortune telling but of Divination—*the introduction of the Divine into the human equation. Divination is often misunderstood as a search for answers as to what will happen, in contrast to what can be <u>willed</u> to happen.*

The greater wisdom and understanding of Man and Universe can be applied first to self-understanding, and second to guiding the self in shaping the future.

The Tarot is much more than a divination system, just as a divination system is much more than fortune telling. And just as hypnosis and particularly self-hypnosis is far more than the stage entertainment that may have been most readers' first exposure to it, just as astrology is very much more than the sun-sign horoscopes appearing in many daily newspapers and popular magazines.

. . . the Tarot is in fact a complete and elaborate system for describing the hidden forces which underlie the universe. It is also the key to all occult science as well as a blueprint for unlocking the various parts of the human psyche. A comprehensive study of the Tarot is a task which is very nearly equal of acquiring a college degree in both psychology and theology. Each Tarot card is an astral mirror of the human mind. Each is also an astral mirror of the human soul.

The New Golden Dawn Ritual Tarot, xi

This duality where the serious function of the subject is carried beneath a popular entertainment function is common to most esoteric sciences. And the reason is simply that of survival.

There is a legend that the wise people of long-ago foresaw a time when the accumulated wisdom of humanity would be suppressed, its books burned, its teachers hunted down, and its truth replaced by dogma, hatred, and avarice. The wise ones asked how they might save the wisdom and preserve it for a time of future enlightenment. They considered secret libraries hidden underground or in great stone structures. They considered small secret societies dedicated to keeping the wisdom hidden in distant retreats. But one wise man suggested that all the knowledge of man and the universe be reduced to symbols which could be portrayed in pictures and used in an ordinary game for entertainment. In this manner, the wisdom would be saved in plain sight and yet always be there to be awakened when mankind would again be ready for the truth. The result is the Tarot, long used as a game, but with the symbols hiding their secrets in plain sight. Thus was the ancient wisdom saved for modern humanity.

Ibid.

Myth and legend contain the secret history of humanity. The art of foresight has always been part of that wisdom, and always has the truth been feared by the rulers and their priests. Now the time has come for revelation and the secrets of the Tarot are exciting the imagination to understand the hidden knowledge. Used for divination, the archetypes pictured on the Major Arcana and the circuitry of their connections and relationships pictured on the Minor Arcana slowly awaken the vast memories in the subconscious mind and the collective unconscious.

In seeking knowledge of the future through the Tarot, the cards release knowledge from the past and present concerning man's relationship to the forces of the universe. Interestingly, although we can only guess at the origins of the Tarot and of the Kabbalah, they "are so strikingly similar in theory that they easily compliment and describe one another. If they indeed came from different origins, it would only serve to prove how universal is the Divine Truth behind them both."*

Thus it is that the Tarot can be used to study the Kabbalah, and the Kabbalah can be used to study the Tarot. And then both can be used in the study of Astrology, and Astrology adds to the study of each. And all three are used in the study of you! Not the 'you' that you were, but the 'you' that you are and the 'you' that you are becoming. The Tarot is the art of your journey through life. Every time you lay the cards out, you have a picture of where you are on that journey.

---

* Chic Cicero & Sandra Tabatha Cicero. *The New Golden Dawn Ritual Tarot,* (Llewellyn, Woodbury, MN, 1991.).

Each card tells a story within a story, and every layout of the cards writes a new chapter in your story.

Each of us is a 'work-in-progress' and it is we, individually, who are in charge of that work. All your relationships, all that happens to you and around you, your job, and all the decisions you make are meaningful parts of the *Great Work* that is your growth and development, *your self-empowerment.*

We will return to the Tarot later in this chapter.

ASTROLOGY—FROM OUTER TO INNER

Astrology, once coeval with astronomy, like the Tarot, also survived largely because of the light entertainment value of sun-sign horoscopes and its simplicity in contrast to the complexity of the necessary calculations for a full horoscope. With the advent of inexpensive computing power, astrology has once again become a scientific method for self-knowledge and understanding, although it has a long ways to go to re-establish its legitimate authority and overcome common misunderstandings.

First of all, astrology does not say that everyone born under a particular sign is more than superficially alike. Astrology is far more complex, and a birth horoscope is calculated to the *exact* time and the *exact* place of birth, and then places the resultant planetary positions in *exact* relationships from which certain conclusions—based on thousands of years of observation—are drawn.

Astrology does not posit a belief that planets project a characteristic force affecting life on earth in particular ways, but rather that every 'body,' including planetary bodies, is surrounded by its own unique energy field that creates a 'resonance' in other fields. At any moment, the field (or aura) surrounding a living creature is a unique coherence of these resonances. At the moment of birth, the newborn life-form's own field is a defined reflection of the field into which it was born—a reflection of each of those resonances as if frozen in time.

It may sound a bit like a confabulation, but think of it this way: One of the first things that the people in the delivery room do is to report the time of birth. One of the next is to take the baby's picture. Now, think if we could take a picture of the baby's astral body—we would see a composite of the energies present at that moment. Then, remembering that the astral is *formative* to the physical: What we see in that astral portrait is the matrix guiding the baby's development forward. That matrix is the same as the 'birth horoscope.' It is like a blueprint. From the birth moment forward, that pattern of energies constantly progresses, and its formative influence is followed developmentally as the baby grows.

We can take another portrait of the astral body at any time, but let's do one for each birthday. That 'birthday horoscope' shows us the energies now developmentally modifying the child's birth horoscope. The birth horoscope is the starting point—nothing can change what we start with, but those changing energies will affect that initial starting pattern.

The birth horoscope and those subsequent pictures tell us about the planetary energies in composite with the earth's energies at the moment and place the astral body is located when the measurements (the astral photograph) are made.

For thousands of years, each planet has been observed, analyzed, and described both individually and in relationship with others, and the concurrent events related both to the individual and the world as a whole recorded. Because of all this data, we have the means to use the birth horoscope for self-understanding and then developmentally for the factors of change.

Together, the horoscope, the Tarot, and the Kabbalah provide the method and structure, along with your daily diary of observation and recording of questions and answers, for true life journaling. You now have the means to take control of your life in the broadest sense possible, for you are working at both the physical and astral (and spiritual) levels.

We will return to interacting with the horoscope later in this chapter.

ASTRAL INTERACTIONS

There are numerous programs we could practice for integrating consciousness and subconsciousness, and hence the physical and the astral, more closely and expanding the conscious awareness of the whole person further, but we want to concentrate on just three in this introduction to the value of such work.

Kabbalistic Path-Working as Guided Meditation

Every pathway has a beginning and an ending: we start at one point, follow a route, and end at another point. Sometimes the only value of the trip is in getting there, or in getting away from the first point, but more often the greater value is in the journey itself. In one of the most creative Kabbalistic techniques, an imaginative journey is taken from one sephirah to another.

There are two ways path-workings are practiced: (1) by a small group of people who usually or at least often work together with one person leading the exercise, or (2) a solitary person who reads descriptions of each of the two sephirah involved, making notes about each, and then launching himself on the journey from the first to the second. Some solitaries and even some groups listen to a recording of the entire journey including descriptions of what that person considers a more-or-less official path-working associated with a particular esoteric order or lodge (not unlike a 'church').

The disadvantage of this latter approach is that the journey is not your own. You want to explore your own subconscious and gain your own understanding of the path and the sephiroth. The advantage, of course, is the voice of experience. The optimum is to do both. You can read or listen to other people's journeys, and you can do your own. A single "trip" is only another small beginning, and the more times you take the trip, the more you will learn.

In every path-working, you are creating a mythic journey; some of these correspond more or less to those of classical mythology while others will involve the same mythical figures but with your participation in *your* version of the story. And that's the point—it is your story in which you are the central character, the hero fulfilling the cosmic drama. Merely reading or hearing or following someone else's story doesn't do as much for organizing your consciousness and for making connections between your experiences and those important universal myths and archetypes.

Think of the difference between reading an adventure story, and playing a computer game in which you are an 'avatar' inside the story. Only in our path-working you know the beginning and the ending and you also understand what you are expected to do but <u>you</u> have to invent the 'how to' of the drama and actually do it.

Look back at the Tree of Life illustration (pg. 121) and start at the bottom. There are three Paths leading upward from Malkuth, the tenth and bottom sephirah, to respectively the ninth, Yesod, directly above, to the eighth, Hod, on the left, and the seventh, Netzach, on the right. The Paths are numbered, and it is the thirty-second path that leads upward to Yesod that should be the first journey.

Traversing the Tree sequentially up from Malkuth is to return home with all the lessons learned, the potentials of the whole person realized, your awareness expanded to the full dimensions of your consciousness and the consciousness from which it is derived.

"The ultimate goal of the Magician is to work through the psychological parts of his/her soul in order to reach the spiritual—the highest unitary level of reality or Source which lies behind all others. The Magician does this by exploring all the levels of reality experimentally—by working his/her way up the Tree of Life by way of personal firsthand experience."*

The Tree of Life maps the creation of the whole universe and of the whole person. We want to traverse the map in reverse to understand and consciously absorb it. You can compare it to an adult returning to his or her childhood haunts to relive those early experiences and see them not only with an adult perspective but with the comprehensive wisdom of the whole human experience tempered with understanding of the whole of creation.

---

* Cicero and Cicero 1991, 160.

Of course you do not yet have that vast awareness, but the totality of the consciousness that is you does, and each exercise of this sort expands your awareness one small step at a time.

The suggested reading list provided at the end of this chapter complements our vision for your ultimate self-empowerment.

MEDITATION AND ASTRAL DOORWAYS
Tarot, Runes, I Ching Hexagrams, Mythology

"Meditation" is word burdened with some confusion. In the Eastern traditions, it more often means *not-thinking* whereas in the Western traditions, it more often means *controlled-thinking*. In various of the Eastern practices, the approach is to silence the thinking mind or to occupy the mind with repetitive chanting of a single sacred word or phrase, again stopping thought. In various of the Western practices the goal is concentration on a single topic and exploring everything about it. In both cases, we have concentration and control over the thinking mind.

Both Eastern and Western traditions include forms of meditation on certain sacred images and the controlled exploration of thoughts engendered by the images, but more often in Eastern practice the meditator expects only to follow established paths while the Western meditator expects to learn something new either in connection with the image or by its aid.

MEDITATION IS SELF-HYPNOSIS

But, East and West do meet on common ground: meditation involves *control* of the thinking process. In the one case, it seems to be an end in itself; in the other, it is a means to an end. In both cases, we are learning something about the mind and we are gaining power in our use of it. We are adding to our self-empowerment.

All hypnosis is self-hypnosis, and meditation is also really self-hypnosis. The preparation for meditation is the same as for self-hypnosis:

Preparation

The goals of meditation are twofold: (1) to calm and control the mind, and (2) to gain knowledge—whether about your self or about a particular matter. This requires that you will be receptive to new ideas and the possibility of overturning old ideas and habits. You are also putting yourself in charge of your life without being dependent upon external authorities. You are becoming self-empowered.

Making Time. Meditation and self-hypnosis are the tools for self-empowerment. Each session should last for thirty minutes or more, and should be repeated daily. This may seem too much of a challenge in your already busy day—but it isn't! One of the most amazing things is that we can always find the time for things that are important. It's a matter of personal organization and scheduling, and knowing that what you accomplish here carries over into your full consciousness and will benefit your whole life.

Security and privacy. Just as with self-hypnosis, you need a location and situation that is secure against disturbance and disruption. Turn off the telephone and other appliances that can interrupt your session. Seat yourself comfortably, but plan not to fall asleep.

Relaxation and Calmness. Proceed with relaxation as you've learned, and put aside all concerns and worries. Be prepared to "hear" words that may be spoken during meditation and allow yourself to respond in inner conversation. Learn from your feelings.

The Question. Unlike your self-hypnosis sessions, you may not be looking for specific answers or accomplished goals, but you are seeking understanding and knowledge. It may be that you are letting a process, like Kabbalistic path-working, teach you about things you have yet to discover. Or it may be that you will use the process to teach you about the Tarot or applications of Astrology.

In many cases, you will be meditating in a continual learning process in which it will prove valuable to review what you previously learned.

In every case, you want a feeling of expectation as you begin the meditation session. You are learning about yourself, about the universe, about big questions and about little questions. As you meditate on a specific image, you are calling upon elements of your consciousness, your body's consciousness, your subconsciousness, your super consciousness, the Akashic Records, the collective unconscious, your spirit guides, the universe, etc. And you are calling upon the image itself, on the whole of which it is a part (as in the case of a single card from a Tarot deck), on its history and evolution, and more.

Write it down. If you do have questions from a previous session, write them in your journal. If you have a specific question about the image for your meditation, write it down. If you have a specific question about anything happening in your life right now, write it down. Through your journal, you are making all these tools with which you are working a part of the whole person you are so that they become "holy" to you.

Visualize it. When meditating upon an image, take it inside to let all your inner powers work on it. Alternately stare at the object and close your eyes to recall it. That part of the session can last for five minutes or so, depending on the object.

ASTRAL DOORWAYS

An astral doorway is the use of an image by a meditator to access information either directly about the image or about an area of the astral world through the subconscious mind. While nearly any image can be used, those that are rich in symbols and correspondences include the Tarot, Runes, I Ching Hexagrams, and various Mythologies. We will illustrate the process using the Tarot but it will be worth your while to continue this practice with astral doorways with these other systems. And following them, you could experiment with the Hebrew letters, Egyptian hieroglyphs, astrological glyphs, etc.

Which Tarot Deck? The first decision you must make is which of the several thousand currently available decks you should use. All useful Tarot Decks today follow a basic pattern established by the Hermetic Order of the Golden Dawn in the late nineteenth century. There are three principal variations of that pattern represented by the

Golden Dawn Ritual Tarot created by Chic and Sandra Tabatha Cicero, the *Rider-Waite Tarot* created by Arthur Edward Waite and Pamela Colman Smith, and the *Thoth Tarot* created by Aleister Crowley and Lady Frieda Harris.

This by no means is intended to suggest that only these three decks are "legitimate," but it is necessary to make the point that the Tarot is based on a specific pattern with Kabbalistic parallels, that the illustrations are not merely pretty pictures but must resonate with a determined set of archetypal images, and it must function for Divination (which is not to be confused with "fortune telling"), in Meditation, as a focus for skrying, and as a symbolic alphabet. All of this requires a substantial conformity with what we might well call the "Golden Dawn Standard" and not a random sequence of pictures intended to amuse, commemorate, celebrate a particular religion, or function as a portable art museum or scrap book.

At the same time, the images on the Tarot should not only fulfill their exact symbolic and Kabbalistic obligations but be pleasing and attractive to the user, excite an energetic response, and "speak" a kind of personal language of style, myth, and even fashion that resonates with the user.

It is not necessary for the cards of every Tarot deck to have the same names—such as "the Lovers," "Chariot" or "Universe," nor that the characters be dressed alike, be racially identical, nor even always gender specific to particular roles, so long as the archetypal obligations are fulfilled.

As you may become more familiar with the Tarot, and decide to use it in divination, you may find the need for several decks to use for specific kinds of readings, just as a good craftsperson will have sets of tools for particular kinds of work. The same personal choices may apply for other uses of the Tarot as in meditation and magical operations. Different decks may express particular philosophical orientations such as environmentally positive, socially active, democratically representative, self-empowering, classless societies; different religious, ethnic, historic, or mythic backgrounds, and so on, as long as these do not interfere with the primary pattern and archetypal reflection.

But, and this is a big exception to previous statement, there is much to be said for the social structure, the specific and timeless images, the specific symbols, the familiar comport and posture of the actors, of the traditional Golden Dawn Tarot family of decks. These were thought out with care and with seeming spiritual guidance to express the inner world principles and not instances of the external reality. They mirror inner realities and have no concern for political correctness now or ever. When they picture wealth it is neither in dollars nor euros but timeless wealth; a Chariot is never a horseless electric hybrid automobile; and the Sun is not hidden behind clouds of pollution.

All these cautions are necessary because almost any set of picture cards are being called "tarot cards" when at best they may function as "oracles" and at worst as a collection of pictures not unlike a collection of baseball cards or pictures of movie stars.

PICK A CARD, ANY CARD

The Tarot's greatest use is as a magickal instrument which can bring spiritual enlightenment to one who studies it. This is because each Tarot card is an astral mirror of the human mind. Meditating on specific cards helps tune the student in to different aspects of his/her own mind establishing a communication link between the conscious and the subconscious. In this manner, imbalances in the personality, which may have gone unnoticed but have caused problems, can be brought to the individual's attention by studying a certain card. These problems can be consciously addressed and spiritual progress may be furthered.

(The New Golden Dawn Ritual Tarot, *159*)

While you might develop a program to study the Tarot cards in some sequence for learning reasons, it is equally valid to start by just choosing a card that 'calls out' to you. Using only the 22 cards of the Major Arcana, look through them until one of them persistently says "Me, I'm the one." It is well, but not necessary, to make that selection in advance of your meditation, leaving it in a place where you may see it several times before your session.

When ready, study the chosen card carefully, both the overall impression and the details. Then stare at it to try to 'burn it into the retina' so that when you close your eyes you can visualize it. It will fade, so you will want to repeat the performance two or three times.

Now, with the card propped up before you, see it as a doorway. You can move back and forth between the real card and the visualized one, but at some point feel yourself moving through the card as a doorway into another world. With your eyes closed, move through the inner landscape, feel yourself at home there, and readily communicate with any person or animal that seeks to talk with you. Do not hurry. Stay awhile right inside the doorway without looking behind yourself.

Pay attention to details. Look at the types and colors of foliage, identify the animals you see, describe the terrain so that you can record this in your journal when you return to the 'home world.' Add to the visual and listen for sounds, touch and feel things, and finally, 'smell the roses.' Try to experience the inner landscape as completely as you normally do the exterior physical landscape.

There's only a bit of caution: This is the astral world, and it is the world of imagination. It is real, but it is also controllable. Nightmares are also real, but they can be scary unless you bring them under control—which you can do. The astral world is one of desire, emotion, and fear. It is imaginary, but your imagination—uncontrolled—can kill you. You can take imaginary trips, but that is not our goal. In using the Tarot card as an astral doorway, you are accepting astral reality as portrayed by the card and as it develops without your interference or guidance. But exercise common sense and caution. If there is a snake in the grass, let it slither away but don't let it bite you. If there is a lion, let it roar, but don't let it eat you. If there is a beautiful person, enjoy the company but don't let him or her talk you into staying in that world or even promising to return.

The astral world is real, but it is not your home world. Your goal is to make it part of your world but not for you to become part of its world. You are neither a tourist or an immigrant. Think of yourself as a student abroad. You are in a foreign land to learn, and then to return home with the benefit of all that you have learned. You have only a student visa, and you are forbidden to immigrate.

Note the similarity between this astral doorway exercise and Kabbalistic path-working: both are well defined. They have a beginning and ending. With the astral doorway, you are to return the way you came. Once you are familiar with the landscape in front of you, turn around and see the backside of the astral doorway you entered and remember that is how you will return home.

Now that you are inside the card, ask yourself questions, or even address them to the people and elements of the card: What do you represent? What are you actually doing? Why these particular colors? What does your clothing signify? Why are you numbered (whatever the card's number)? Why are you named (whatever the card name is)? Why is the Hebrew letter (whatever the letter is) assigned to you? Why is the astrological symbol (whatever it is) assigned to you? And so on. You may hear answers or only feel answers, or maybe you will have to come back another time.

When you feel your time is up, turn around and go back through the astral door. Pull yourself together and feel your physical self. Enjoy a cup of coffee or tea or other nonalcoholic beverage. And record your experience in your journal, including the answers to your questions. Decide what you've learned about yourself and about the astral world.

Finally, pick another card for your next visit.

It is also desirable to add a certain ritual structure to your astral journeys. It doesn't have to be complex and rigid, but the point is to firmly establish the demarcation between this world and that—so visualizing an actual door or curtain with the image of the chosen card or symbol emblazed on the front side, and the reverse of the same image on the back side is an easy start. Carrying an imaginary voice recorder into which you speak of your impressions and from which you will make notes after you return through that same doorway— that you firmly close behind you—is another. Another simple idea is to have a real cane or wand in this world with an imagined duplicate that you carry when in the other world is a further simple step.

RESTORING UNITY

We are not just learning things *about* the Tarot or the Kabbalah, but we are reuniting inner and outer, astral and physical, conscious and subconscious. The key element, however, is your goal of self-empowerment—meaning that you are in control of your imagination, your emotions, your thoughts, while recognizing the unity of all.

Eons ago, it is believed by some occultists and philosophers that we were astral beings only, and then slowly we became involved in the physical world. For a long time our astral and physical experiences were united. Then we lost that duality and have the present separation. As astral beings, our behavior was instinctual and our relationship to Nature was 'natural.' Now, our job is to reverse the experience and reunite with the astral, and later with the other planes to expand our conscious awareness of the totality of the whole person we are and the whole universe we live within. Your self-empowerment is founded on this growing experience of the greater whole.

ASTRAL PROJECTION AND ASTRAL TRAVEL

First we have to clear up a matter of confusion and common mis-definition.

What is generally called the out-of-body experience is not astral projection, but is the projection of the etheric body, the energy matrix of the physical body. It is part of the physical plane, and hence functions in the physical world with some degree of physical interaction. On the other hand, it is not a dense physical body so it can pass through closed doors, speed off to another physical location, and observe what people are doing.

It's what most people think of when "astral projection" is mentioned. And it is an out-of-body experience. The etheric body does have limitations, however, and can be subjected to energy stresses that will react upon the physical body. It cannot function on the astral plane because it truly is part of the physical body, or the physical/etheric body as these two are always joined together (via the silver cord) so long as the physical body is alive.

It is etheric projection that sometimes occurs spontaneously when the physical body is weak, or when it is anesthetized, or suddenly released at death to appear before a loved one. And it is the etheric body that can be involved in *shape shifting* and as an *etheric revenant*. Here we have two of the most interesting of paranormal phenomena long part of folklore and the basis for much horror fiction.

In shape shifting, the etheric body is molded into the shape of another human or more commonly into an animal as in lyncanthropy (werewolf). An etheric revenant is the continued use of the etheric body after the death of the physical by means of the intent and desire of the person aided by special rituals and (1) the preservation of the physical body (embalmed) and its protection from disturbance (burial in a special place), (2) its protection from sunlight, and (3) its regular nourishment with a source of etheric energies (like blood). Sound familiar? Vampires never die. And folklore never lies.

Astral projection is not, technically, an out-of-body experience but rather a state of consciousness that may include the creation of a thought form of astral 'substance,' which can act as a vehicle for movement in the astral world. This is not a matter of moving in space, at least not in dimensional space, but in consciousness—or, if you prefer, in Spirit. *Where Thou art, there I AM.*

At one extreme, this can be experienced as mystical ecstasy.

The two main methods of the traditional and esoteric Kabbalah are meditation (yoga) and practical Kabbalah (magic). By Yoga is meant that rigorous system of mental and self-discipline which has as its primary aim the absolute and complete control of the thinking principle, the Ruach; the ultimate object being to obtain the faculty with which to still the stream of thought at will, so that which is behind (as it were), or above, or beyond the mind can manifest on to the stillness thus produced. The quiescence of the mental turbulence is the primary essential. With this faculty

> *at command, the student is taught to exalt the mind by the various technical methods of magick until it overrides the normal limitations and barriers of its nature, ascending in a tremendous unquenchable column of fire-like ecstasy to the universal consciousness, with which it becomes united. Once having become at one with transcendental existence, it intuitively partakes of universal knowledge, which is considered to be a more reliable source of information than the rational introspection of the intellect or the experimental scientific investigation of matter can give.*
>
> (A Garden of Pomegranates, *20*)

At the other extreme, astral projection is simply an act of imagination—remembering that what is imagined is real. In a "Body of Light" (created from the 'astral light' substance), you can explore the different reality of the astral world. Even though there is astral 'substance'—the astral light—this world is nonspatial and yet is everywhere. It is perceived through a switch in consciousness. While nonspatial in our usual sense, it has the features of a landscape. It is an interior world with many of the characteristics of the exterior world.

And, we have to keep reminding ourselves that the astral world is our own subconscious. As we explore the astral and as we learn to understand its rules and laws, mapping its geography, noting similarities and differences to the exterior world, we are mapping and learning about our subconsciousness. We are discovering the reality of Inner and Outer, becoming as aware of the subconscious as we are of the conscious, perceiving unity without loss of duality and with ourselves making a trinity and thus Wholeness.

YOU AND YOUR HOROSCOPE

It's one thing to talk about astrology and the value of a real horoscope drawn to the exact time and place of birth, and another thing altogether to bring home its objective power for self-understanding. This is not a "commercial," but the most practical and least expensive way to experience this is with a computer-generated chart and written horoscope interpretation. We've recommended one in the suggested reading list at the end of the chapter.

Your own horoscope allows you see the tool and experience its benefit. The goal of self-empowerment begins with self-understanding.

SUGGESTED READING

Kabbalah

Christopher, Liam Thomas. *Kabbalah, Magic and the Great Work of Self-Transformation.*Woodbury, MN: Llewellyn Worldwide, 2006.

Godwin, David. *Godwin's Cabalistic Encyclopedia.* Woodbury, MN: Llewellyn Worldwide, 1994.

Regardie, Israel. *A Garden of Pomegranates*, 3rd edition with new material by Chic and Sandra Cicero. Woodbury, MN: Llewellyn Worldwide, 1999.

————. *The Middle Pillar*, 3rd edition with new material by Chic and Sandra Cicero. Woodbury, MN: Llewellyn Worldwide, 1998.

Tarot

Cicero, Chic and Sandra. *The New Golden Dawn Ritual Tarot.* Woodbury, MN: Llewellyn Worldwide, 1991.

Louis, Anthony. *Tarot Plain & Simple.* Woodbury, MN: Llewellyn Worldwide, 1996.

Tyson, Donald. *1-2-3 Tarot.* Woodbury, MN: Llewellyn Worldwide, 2004.

Tarot Decks

Go to www.llewellyn.com, and then to Tarot & Divination for a catalog of Tarot Decks.

Astral Projection

Denning, Melita, and Osborne Phillips. *Practical Guide to Astral Projection.* Woodbury, MN: Llewellyn Worldwide, 2001.

Tyson, Donald. *Soul Flight.* Woodbury, MN: Llewellyn Worldwide, 2007.

Astrology

George, Llewellyn. *Llewellyn's New A to Z Horoscope Maker & Interpreter*. Woodbury, MN: Llewellyn Worldwide, 2003.

Llewellyn's Astrology Reports—*AstroTalk Detailed Chart Analysis #APS03.525 U.S.$20.00. Go to www.llewellyn.com/bookstore/astrology_readings.bhp with your exact birthtime, date, year and place of birth.*

CHAPTER SEVEN

THE PROOF
IS IN THE PUDDING

Case studies from thirty years of practice and research directed by
Dr. Joe H. Slate, Emeritus Professor of Psychology at Athens State
University, Athens, Alabama

Nothing offers more convincing evidence of the power of self-hypnosis than firsthand examples. Case studies of personal experiences have repeatedly shown the remarkable capacity of self-hypnosis to empower mentally, physically, and spiritually. They demonstrate with clarity the vast range of possibilities now available to everyone through self-hypnosis.

The case studies that follow illustrate a variety of self-hypnosis programs and goal-related applications. The subjects (people) of the studies presented here set their own goals and then selected a self-hypnosis program that seemed appropriate to those goals. They personally tailored the program to fit their preferences and needs while retaining its four essential elements: (1) a clear statement of goals; (2) positive affirmations of success; (3) relevant visualization; and (4) post-hypnotic suggestion.

Studying these case reports will facilitate your greater understanding of the process and your ability to develop your own programs.

The clear statement of goals was formulated prior to the trance induction and restated upon reaching the successful trance state. The positive affirmations of success accompanied by relevant visualization were presented during the hypnotic state. The post-hypnotic suggestion designed to establish a cue for later use in activating the effects of the trance experience was presented immediately prior to exiting the trance state.

The cases, chosen from a large collection, were selected because they illustrate the power of self hypnosis to make genuine improvements in personal life in simple and fundamental ways. The examples are familiar so as not to challenge the reader with cutting-edge cases of dramatic cures or astonishing new skills. Ordinary life is filled with many opportunities for self-improvement and with improvement comes self-empowerment. Self-improvement is preceded by self-understanding and recognition of needs and inadequacies. Every act of self-understanding and self-improvement is a step forward in your self-empowerment in which you have chosen to be the master of your fate and to control your destiny.

CASE STUDY 1: GEESE IN FLIGHT
Overcoming Feelings of Inferiority and Compulsive Shopping

This real estate broker, age 28, has an impressive history of career success and community service. Beneath the surface, however, she struggled since early childhood with deep feelings of inferiority that she attributes, at least in part, to an impoverished background. She attempted to compensate for her mounting feelings of inadequacy through her superior academic performance as a college student, and then later on, through her career achievements and community activities. She became an active participant in projects related to environmental protection, animal rights, historical preservation, and community beautification. Along another line, she became a compulsive shopper, especially for shoes. She, in fact, accumulated over the years dozens upon dozens of pairs of shoes, many of which she kept in their original boxes. Unfortunately, her feelings of inferiority only worsened. They, in fact, seemed to have taken on a life of their own, draining her of energy like a parasitic vampire.

Finally, her long struggle to overcome the deepening feelings of inferiority took an unexpected turn when, in a recurring dream, she observed geese migrating in a distinct "V" formation over a mountain range in the light of a full moon. The vivid dream was especially relevant because of her active participation in animal rights and her profound commitment to protecting endangered species and their habitats. Accompanying each recurring dream was a deep sense of peace and well-being.

Inspired by the dream experience, she decided to use self-hypnosis in her effort to overcome the persistent feelings of inferiority. As a former student with training in hypnosis, she used a variation of the eye fixation program in which she focused on a shiny object situated slightly above eye-level to induce the trance state. Upon reaching successful trance, she affirmed her goal of becoming empowered with feelings of adequacy, self-worth, and security. Almost instantly, a highly detailed image of herself as a second grade student seated at her desk unfolded clearly before her. As the image emerged, her attention was drawn to her shoe where the tip of a toe had worn through. Embarrassed by the sight, she concealed the damaged shoe with the exposed toe as best she could by resting her other shoe over it.

As the dream image slowly faded, her attention spontaneously shifted from the classroom to the familiar flock of geese migrating over a mountain range in a perfect "V" formation against a full moon, exactly as in her recurring dream. Suddenly, she experienced a magical oneness with the waterfowl and a total lifting of the negative baggage of inferiority that had distressed her since childhood. Empowered by the experience, she concluded the trance with the post-hypnotic suggestion that by simply visualizing geese migrating against a full moon, she would instantly replace any residual feelings of inferiority with a powerful sense of security and worth.

Through the combination of an inspiring dream and self-hypnosis, she successfully banished the deep-seated feelings of inferiority and replaced them with a profound awareness of personal significance that gave new meaning and happiness to her life. Her compulsion for shopping, especially for shoes, likewise vanished. She discovered for herself the best of all personal therapists—the one existing deep within.

CASE STUDY 2: A HEALING NATURE TRAIL
Overcoming Chronic Abdominal Pain

This 24-year-old male science teacher had a long history of severe bloating accompanied by stabbing abdominal pain. His social functions were interrupted and he frequently missed work because of flare-ups. He had seen several specialists and tried various prescribed medications, but nothing proved effective, and the side effects of medication posed a serious problem. He decided to use self-hypnosis in a last-ditch effort to alleviate the physical symptoms along with the stress and anxiety associated with the condition.

To induce the trance state, he used a variation of the interactive relaxation program in which he mentally relaxed his body, focusing first on the muscles in his forehead and then progressing slowly downward. Once in a deeply relaxed state, he used reverse counting interspersed with suggestions of depth and drowsiness to induce hypnosis. Upon achieving successful hypnosis, he visualized a dense forest with a nature trail winding through it. He imagined walking along the trail and absorbing throughout his body its bright healing energies.

He then visualized his digestive system as, like the nature trail, aglow with radiant healing energy. He accompanied the "inner healing imagery," as he called it, with powerful affirmations of health, relaxation, and freedom from the severe bloating and severe pain that had plagued him for many years and worsened at times of stress. He concluded the program with the post-hypnotic suggestion that by simply visualizing the nature trail, he would become instantly relaxed and infused with radiant healing energy deep within.

The rewards of the program, by his report, were immediate. Within a few weeks of daily practice and frequent use of the post-hypnotic visualization cue, he experienced a significant reduction of painful symptoms along with marked improvements in the overall quality of his daily life.

This case study of a young teacher illustrates the complex connection between mind and body and our capacity to influence it through self-hypnosis. At this very moment, your subconscious healing resources beckon your awareness and invite your interaction. Through self-hypnosis, you can activate and target them on your personal health goals. The results are an energized, enriched, and empowered life.

CASE STUDY 3: SELF-HYPNOSIS AND SLEEP LEARNING

Becoming Proficient in German

This 27-year-old doctoral student in clinical psychology had successfully completed most of the stringent requirements for her Ph.D. degree. Only one major hurdle remained—a competency examination showing a reading proficiency in German. Unfortunately, she had no background in that language. In preparation for the examination, which required translating a scholarly German writing into English, she used a three-pronged approach that included private tutoring in German, self-hypnosis, and sleep learning, each designed to accelerate a reading mastery of the language.

Having participated as an undergraduate student in our early laboratory research on self-hypnosis at the University of Alabama that included various sleep-arrest programs, she decided to use a finger-spread induction approach. For that approach, the fingers of either hand are held in a tense, finger-spread position during the drowsy state to induce hypnosis immediately preceding sleep. Upon reaching the pre-sleep hypnotic state with the fingers remaining in the spread position, she presented a brief dialogue that included the following affirmations:

I AM endowed with the ability to learn German.

I AM committed to develop that ability.

I will use sleep to acquire a reading competency in German.

My dreams will work with me as I work with them to achieve this goal.

Upon relaxing my hand, I will enter restful sleep, during which my mastery of German will rapidly advance.

Upon completing the dialogue and before falling asleep, she visualized a symbol of her success: the Ph.D. diploma with her name inscribed upon it. She then relaxed her hand as peaceful sleep ensued.

Throughout her repeated use of the program, she regularly experienced dreams of reading in German, to include passages from Wilhelm Wundt's noted work, *An Introduction to Psychology*. In record time, she acquired a reading competency in German. When she later reported to the test center at the appointed time for the proficiency examination, the German book presented to her for translation into English was, to her amazement, the familiar book she had seen frequently in her dreams—*An Introduction to Psychology* by Wilhelm Wundt. She passed the exam with an excellent rating.

This student's experience, in which self-hypnosis combined with sleep and dreaming seemed to work together in promoting learning, raises several interesting questions. First and foremost, can sleep when directed toward specific goals actually accelerate learning? Can self-hypnosis activate a specific subconscious faculty related to a particular intellectual skill, such as learning a new language? Can sleep and dreaming actually involve precisely the faculties required for mastering a particular skill? Can dreams activate certain psychic faculties related to a specific goal striving? Along that line, was this student's dream of reading from a particular book merely a chance happening, or was there instead a subconscious precognitive faculty at work? Could a language skill unavailable to consciousness exist full-blown in the subconscious, perhaps a language acquired during a past lifetime? Since we do not know all there is to know about the powers of the mind, perhaps the most rational answer to these searching questions is yet another question: *Why not?*

CASE STUDY 4: BLOOD ON THE FLOOR
Past Life Regression to Discover the Source of Irrational Fear

A phobia can be defined as a persistent fear of objects or situations for which actual danger either does not exist or is magnified beyond reasonable proportions. Among the most common are (1) acrophobia—fear of high places; (2) astraphobia—irrational fear of storms, thunder, and lightning; (3) claustrophobia—paralyzing reaction to enclosed places; (4) hematophobia—fear and reaction to blood, (5) monophobia—exaggerated fear of being alone; (6) mysophobia—fear of contamination or germs; and (7) zoophobia—fear of animals or a particular animal.

Phobias seem to be far more common among adolescents and young adults, possibly due to the adjustment demands and stress often characteristic to these age groups. Regardless of age factors, persons with phobias usually admit that they either have no logical reason to be afraid or that a reasonable cause must exist but somewhere beyond their conscious awareness. That unknown cause, once uncovered, can give rationality to an otherwise irrational fear and, in many instances, extinguish it altogether, at times in an instant.

The capacity of enlightenment to extinguish irrational fear was dramatically illustrated by a college student whose persistent fear of blood seriously restricted her life. Even when the probability of being exposed to blood was remote, she remained fearful that a condition could arise in which she would either view blood or be exposed in some other way to it. Such a situation did in fact arise during a classroom presentation of a film on drug addiction, which included a segment on intravenous injection during which blood trickled down the arm. The experience was so distressful that she quickly left the room.

As a result of the experience, she volunteered to participate in the University's research on altered states of consciousness that included the development of a past-life regression program called EM-RC, an acronym for eye-movement/reverse counting (Slate 2008). She quickly mastered the self-induction program and used it to uncover the source of her fear of blood.

As it turns out, she discovered through past-life regression that she had been the daughter of a prominent plantation owner in southeastern Tennessee during the Civil War. Her fiancé, a Confederate soldier, sustained a serious gunshot injury to the chest in a nearby battle with Federal troops and was rushed to the plantation mansion where a temporary hospital had been set up. Unfortunately, soon after his arrival at the mansion, he collapsed upon the floor before a fireplace in an upstairs bedroom. She rushed to his side as he bled profusely from the deep wound. Soaked in his blood, she held him in her arms until, within minutes, he was dead.

Upon exiting the trance state, she knew at once the source of the fear of blood that had tormented her for many years. She also knew that her fear of blood had been, in an instant, totally extinguished. She had discovered for herself the liberating power of past-life enlightenment.

The impact of past life regression for this student was so profound that she felt compelled to research the experience. She found through her review of Civil War archives that a historic antebellum mansion resembling the one she had seen during regression still stands in a remote area of southeastern Tennessee where a well-known battle had occurred. She promptly contacted the mansion's current owner and arranged a visit of the historic site. Upon viewing the columned mansion from a distance, she experienced a powerful sense of déjà vu that became even stronger as she neared the building. Accompanied by the owner, she toured the eerily familiar mansion room by room. Finally, upon entering a second-floor bedroom, her attention was drawn to a darkened blood stain on the old wood floor before an open fireplace. The mansion's owner explained that, despite all efforts to remove it, the stain had been there since the Civil War.

This former student is today a prominent psychotherapist in private practice. Her specialty is the treatment of anxiety disorders through past life regression.

CASE STUDY 5: STOP SMOKING NOW

The Cure of an Addiction

Possibly nothing more vividly illustrates the power of mind over body than the self-hypnosis programs that break the smoking habit. The most successful quit smoking programs recognize that power and the effectiveness of the "all or nothing" approach in which the smoking habit is instantly extinguished. That approach was illustrated by an undergraduate college student, age 22, who had begun smoking at age 14 and soon increased his tobacco use to an average of two packs daily. In partial fulfillment of a parapsychology course requirement, he designed a research project to test for himself the effectiveness of self-hypnosis in breaking his smoking habit. The program included the essential elements of self-hypnosis along with an aversive conditioning situation in which he used a noxious mental stimulus to suppress an unwanted behavior. In this situation, the noxious stimulus was self-induced nausea and the unwanted behavior was smoking.

The setting for the experiment was a controlled laboratory setting free of distractions. While resting comfortably in a seated position, he used the upward gaze followed by reverse counting and suggestions of relaxation to induce a successful hypnotic state. To test his receptiveness to suggestion, he used hand anesthesia to remove all feeling from his hand and then return it. Next, he stated his goal as follows: *"Beginning now, I AM a nonsmoker. The need to smoke is now replaced with the satisfaction of being a nonsmoker. From this moment forward, any thought of smoking will be met with the discomfort of nausea followed by a powerful image of the word NO in bold block letters."* As the trance state continued, he tested the effectiveness of his suggestions by visualizing himself taking a cigarette from a pack and preparing to light it. As the image unfolded, he experienced nausea so severe that he became concerned that he was about to vomit. Upon putting the cigarette aside, the word NO appeared boldly before him and the nausea ceased. He then affirmed with confidence, "I AM now a nonsmoker."

He concluded the trance state with a restatement of the post-hypnotic suggestion that any thought of smoking would be met with the discomfort of nausea followed by a clear mental image of the word NO.

This former student is today a practicing psychologist whose orientation is cognitive-behaviorist. Clinical hypnosis is a major component of his highly successful practice. Thanks to his innovative research project as an undergraduate student in parapsychology, he remains a nonsmoker. In his opinion, the word "no" in proper context is one of the most powerful words in the English language

CASE STUDY 6: A GROUP STUDY OF LEARNING AND MEMORY

The Secret of Learning, Memory, and Empowerment

Learning can be defined as changes in thoughts, feelings, and/or behaviors resulting from practice and experience. Memory can be defined as the retention of those changes. Underlying both learning and memory are, however, complex mental processes, each of which interacts with the other. Fortunately, self-hypnosis programs are now available to intervene into those processes in ways that improve both learning and memory.

One of the most effective programs designed specifically to achieve that goal is called Learning and Memory Empowerment, a self-hypnosis program developed in our labs at Athens State University. It's an easily administered program that begins with a stated objective related to learning and memory. The trance state is then induced through hand levitation in which either hand, resting lightly on the thighs, is allowed to rise gently to the forehead as suggestions of drowsiness and relaxation are presented. Upon touching the forehead, the hand is allowed to slowly return to the rest position as suggestions of going deeper and deeper into hypnosis are presented. Deepening suggestions, including reverse counting, are then presented as needed. Once the desired depth of hypnosis is attained, affirmations related to improving learning and memory are presented. Here are a few examples: *I AM at my mental peak; I AM empowered to learn rapidly and remember clearly; My mind is clear and free of distractions; I AM now in command of the powers within;* and *The knowledge I need is now available to me.* The trance state is concluded with the post-hypnotic suggestion that simply touching the temple with either hand will instantly activate the highest mental functions related to learning and memory. The "temple touch" as it's called thus becomes a post-hypnotic cue which can then be used on demand at any time.

This case study, rather than an individual study, is a group study of 27 college students enrolled in an experimental parapsychology course at Athens State University. At midpoint of the course, Learning and Memory Empowerment was introduced by the instructor, first as a group activity, and then for independent use by each student. Students were encouraged to practice the self-hypnosis program at least once weekly and then to use the post-hypnotic cue of touching the temple as often as needed, to include during weekly course examinations.

Assessment of the study's results included self-evaluations by each student along with comparisons of student test scores before and after the introduction of the self-hypnosis program. This two-pronged assessment revealed significant improvements in both learning and memory for each student following the introduction of self-hypnosis. Students, without exception, rated the self-hypnosis program as effective, a finding confirmed by objective course evaluations.

Our follow-on studies found that many of the students who participated in this research continued to use the self-hypnosis program, including the temple touch cue, in other college courses as well as later on in their careers. As one former student put it, "It's a skill I'll use for a lifetime."

This group study suggests once again that *complexity seeks simplicity.* Our most complex mental functions, including those existing in the subconscious, seek not only our conscious awareness but our application as well. Learning and Memory Empowerment is a highly practical, easily mastered self-hypnosis program that empowers you to activate the intricate mental processes required to increase your command of new knowledge and to use it as needed. Who could ask for more than that?

REFERENCE

Slate, Joe H. *Beyond Reincarnation: Experience Your Past Lives & Lives Between Lives.* Woodbury, MN: Llewellyn Worldwide, 2008.

CHAPTER EIGHT

THE FINAL CHAPTER

Of course there is no "final chapter" on this subject of self-empowerment. There can't be, for we humans are 'a work in process,' and when that process is completed for all of us, everything will end. And then, I believe it starts over again, but at some higher dimension.

I don't believe humans can ever know everything, and hence no one can write a final chapter to a book on our continuing evolution. We're here to grow into the Whole Person we're supposed to be, and that includes a role as a 'co-creator' of the ever growing and evolving universe as we know it in ways we possibly never will understand.

This is a book on self-empowerment and about the use of self-hypnosis in programs of self-improvement, self-healing, self-discovery, and understanding the nature and functions of the subconscious.

"Self-empowerment" is simply bringing the Self (big "S") into full development as the whole person you were born to be. It sounds grand, and it is. It's more than we can even dream of being—but it's all there, laid out from the beginning as a matrix guiding our continuous growth and development. From a universal beginning each of us has become a unique individual growing and working to fulfill all our potential in unique ways that contribute to the whole of all there is.

It's not 'fated' because everything is still evolving for that too is part of the great plan. You are destined for greatness, and when you accept that and believe in it, more opportunities for growth will open before you. We rarely understand them as such, but try to see everything in this light and see everything as an opportunity.

"Self-empowerment" must not be confused with being 'selfish' or with being oblivious to the needs of others. The more empowered you become, the more will you relate positively with others and the more will your actions—no matter how seemingly minor—be of benefit to the greater scheme of things.

Our ability to grow and develop our individual selves in unique expressions is as important as is our ability to discover and develop common interests with others. *Nature abhors 'sameness' in the same way She abhors a vacuum!* Look about you and be amazed at the diversity of life-forms while remembering that the visible part of the spectrum is just a small portion of the whole that is explored as we extend our vision microscopically and then telescopically. And then extend that vision still further as we explore other dimensions of the astral, mental, and spiritual worlds.

Next take any of those individual expressions of diversity—perhaps conveniently starting with another person with whom you have close relationship and then on to other people, and then to pets and on to other birds, animals, and fish, where you have a chance to distinguish the uniqueness that separates each entity from the species as a whole. Use your imagination to move on into invisible realms and understand that even particles of the same substance have uniqueness as well as sameness. No matter how large or how small, how dense or how subtle, or how near or far, there is diversity and commonality within the whole.

It all may sound like a bunch of platitudes—but it isn't. The big "S" Self knows how small each of us is, but also just how much bigger the role we play is. It's a grand adventure, the biggest game of all, the finest role you'll ever play, and the most important job you will ever have.

But, look once again at the title, *Self-Empowerment through Self-Hypnosis*. Through self-hypnosis you are empowering your self. Self-hypnosis is just a technique, and a very efficient one, we are using to enable you to do for yourself things that no one else can do for you. Certainly there are many good teachers you can learn from and many good books that you can benefit from; there are many counselors and others who want to help and who can help along the way—but—

ultimately it's all in your hands: *you have to pull it together and you have to take the final steps yourself.*

And even that is not final! Think of the Aquarian Man who corresponds to the Star Tarot Card—the Man or Woman beneath the stars pouring healing water upon the earth beneath: Man channeling beneficence from Heaven to Earth. The more empowered we become, the more beneficence flows through us. This is the symbol and the call of the New Aquarian Age. We are co-creators and part of the process. It is only as self-empowered human beings that we fulfill our roles as co-creators in service to the Greater Whole.

In an earlier discussion of the Kabbalah, we quoted:

The Universe began not with an atom or a subatomic particle, but with a thought in the mind of God. This thought of Creation encompassed a world in which every human being would enjoy happiness and fulfillment, free from any form of chaos or pain. This is what the Creator desires and intends.

But bringing about the realization of the Creator's desire is up to us. For the manifestation of complex fulfillment to take place, we need to evolve into our truest, greatest selves. In our thoughts, our feelings, and our actions, we need to erase negativity and replace darkness with Light. It is for this purpose that the teachings and tools of Kabbalah were given to all humanity.

By Rav Berg in the Introduction to *The Sacred Zohar*, The Kabbalah Center, Los Angles (2007).

As my co-author wrote:

INTERDIMENSIONAL INTERACTION PROGRAM

"In recent years, self-hypnosis has progressively gained recognition as a highly practical and effective approach for accessing the subconscious, activating its dormant potentials, and focusing them on designated goals. The applications of self-hypnosis are, in fact, so extensive that the limits, assuming they exist in the first place, are yet to be defined. You can, in fact, use self-hypnosis to discover—and in some instances generate—totally new powers within yourself while increasing

your effectiveness in using them to empower your life (Slate 2001)."
Self-hypnosis is one of the most powerful options known for accelerating your personal growth and actualizing your highest potentials.

"Nothing more clearly illustrates our spiritual essence than our
capacity to interact with the spirit dimension. Our awareness of spirit
guides and in some instances, the departed, illustrates our capacity as
spiritual beings to interact with the spiritual realm. To explore that
interaction and its empowering potentials, the Interdimensional Interaction Program was formed at Athens State University under the
auspices of the Foundation. A major objective of the program was
to determine the relevance of self-hypnosis to spirituality, to include
mediumistic communications."

Such empowerment cannot be bought and comes, not as a gift, but
through self-discovery and understanding, and then through self-development of the powers innate to the whole person. As you gain knowledge of self, that knowledge—and the power to use it—flows into self.
Such power is natural and evolutionary but, historically, it has been
suppressed through the denial of knowledge about self and the potentials of the whole person. And the opportunities for personal growth
and self-empowerment were limited by all the challenges to individual
and group survival in the pre-industrial ages.

Now, despite cyclical distortions in our economic growth, more
people have choices between spending their surplus on houses with
more rooms than they need and cars with more horsepower than
can safely be used, and nations can choose between wasteful military adventures and wider investments in economic development
so that young men and women have better things to do than killing
each other under the tutelage of self-anointed spokespersons for God
teaching that hate rather than love is the Word of the Creator.

It need not be that way!

*Self-hypnosis provides a new generation of people with the power to
facilitate the most exciting moment in human history: the true transition from other-directed Piscean Man to inner-directed Aquarian Man.*

I promised a surprise answer to the question of "Just WHO do you think you are?" The *true you* is without describable characteristics because this you is *pure consciousness.* That's who, or what, you really are: *pure consciousness* on a journey through life, a tiny bit of the universal consciousness that is the inner Divinity that empowers every one of us.

You, I, all of us have the power to change the world as we know it. Each of us can invest in personal growth and the development of our potentials as whole persons able to work together and through the inner structure of the universe to mend the world's wounds.

That's the ultimate meaning of self-empowerment.

You probably bought this book in anticipation of the practical and spiritual applications of self-hypnosis—and that is what you have. But you now also have the skills to move on to ever greater things. Your expanding awareness will provide opportunities for success in all your ventures.

—Carl Llewellyn Weschcke
December 21, 2008

Glossary and Suggested Reading

Terms and Resources Related to Self-Empowerment and Self-Hypnosis

While this Glossary is neither a dictionary nor an encyclopedia, it does contain elements of both. Most of the definitions given here are specific to words as used in this book, although we have included others of interest to the study of self-empowerment and self-hypnosis, and included references to the Kabbalah, Astrology, and the Tarot intended to give the reader a solid base for further study and practice. For this reason, the first words after the search word explain the context. In some cases, references are suggested to the reader for further research on the subject involved.

Abyss. (Kabbalah—Tree of Life) A division on the Tree of Life separating the top three sephiroth from the rest of the Tree. A separation of the noumenal from the phenomenal.

Affirmations. (Self-Hypnosis) As used in Self-Hypnosis, these are positive assertions of that which is desired as if it is already realized. This is vital to the involvement of the subconscious mind.

Ain. (Kabbalah—Tree of Life) "Naothing." It is the outermost of the three veils of negative existence above the Tree of Life.

Ain Soph. (Kabbalah—Tree of Life) "Limitless." The middle of the three veils of negative existence.

Ain Soph Aur. (Kabbalah—Tree of Life) "Limitless Light." The innermost of the three veils of negative existence preceding Kether.

Ajna. (Etheric Body) The 'third eye' chakra, located at the brow, color indigo, associated planet Moon, associated sephiroth Chokmah and Binah.

Akasha. The element of Spirit, one of the five tattvas or elemental forces—the others being Air, Fire, Water, and Earth, which are derived from Spirit. It is symbolized by an indigo egg shape.

Akashic Records. The collective unconscious is a kind of group mind that is inherited from all our ancestors and includes all the memories and knowledge acquired by humans and sometimes is called 'the Akashic Records.' It is believed to exist on the higher astral and lower mental planes and to be accessible by the super consciousness through the subconscious mind in deep trance states induced through hypnosis, self-hypnosis, meditation, and guided meditation. It is a function of the Astral Light to retain all that has ever happened in thought and deed.

Alpha Level. The beta state of ordinary alertness and concentrated mental activity typically ranges from 14 to 22 Hz. The alpha or relaxed wakefulness state can range from brainwave levels of 8 to 14 Hz. You can easily induce the alpha state by simply settling back, closing your eyes, and rolling your eyeballs gently upward. The theta state of drowsiness and dreaming can range from levels of 4 to 8 Hz, whereas the deepest stages of sleep can range from 0.5 to 4 Hz.

Altered State of Consciousness (ASC). Wakefulness and sleep are the two most familiar states of consciousness. Others include dreaming, meditation, trance, hypnosis and self-hypnosis, hallucination, astral projection, etc. ASCs can be induced by sleep deprivation, chanting, fasting, ecstatic dancing, drumming, sex, psychedelic drugs, and conscious self-programming. Once you've been 'there,' it is easier to get there again.

Anahata. (Etheric Body) The chakra located at the heart, color green, associated planet Sun or Venus, associated sephirah Tiphareth.

Analytic Psychology. Jungian Psychology, which see.

Anima. The Woman in every man. In Jung's psychology, it is the mythic ideal of the feminine that a man projects onto women. It manifests in fantasy, romance, sexual behavior, the estrogen hormone, and in feminine energy.

Anima Mundi. The "Soul of the World." There has been a dual usage for this phrase: (1) As the World Mind or Global Consciousness, divided into *spiritus mundi* or world vital force and *corpus mundi* or the world physical body; (2) The divine essence that permeates everything, also known as Astral Light, Prana, Animal Magnetism, Spirit.

Animal Magnetism. Etheric, or life, energy that, like Reich's *Orgone,* is present in all animal life. It can be concentrated, stored, transferred and projected by magical practices—essentially the use of a trained imagination. It formed the basis for many of the practices of *mesmerism,* considered by some to be an early forerunner of Hypnotism.

Animus. The Man in every woman. In Jung's psychology, it is the mythic ideal of the masculine that a woman projects onto men. It manifests in fantasy, romance, sexual response, the testosterone hormone, and in masculine energy.

Apas. The Tattwa of elemental Water. It is symbolized by a silver crescent with the horns pointing upward as if a container.

Application Programs. The aptitudes and capabilities you demonstrate. Many self-improvement classes give you new aptitudes that augment your Application Programs.

Aquarian Age. (Astrology) The zodiacal age of approximately 2,150 years length subsequent to the Piscean Age. The 'spirit' of these Ages is believed to be characterized by symbolism and general astrological characteristics of the zodiacal sign. As the Piscean Age is identified as the age of Christianity (and its authoritarian origins and offshoots), the Aquarian Age is associated with the "New Age," which Carl Jung believed to have begun in 1940. The general association ascribed to Aquarius is that this will be the Age of Man, of Intellect rather than Emotion, and of self-responsibility rather than the 'shepherd's crook.' Fish swim in a collective 'school,' while Man walks alone.

While the ending of an age and the beginning of another is theoretically well determined by the astronomical position of the Sun at the Spring Equinox, even that is debated as occurring in a range from 2012 to 2374. As a practical matter, like "morning" or "evening," the transition between zodiacal ages is indefinite.

Archetypes. (Tarot) A universal image and center of psychological function and energy mostly similar across nationalities, races, cultures, and historical times. Generally speaking, "Mom" is the same mom everywhere. Nevertheless, there may be some minor variation across long established cultures as expressed in dominant religions, and personal variants may be the source of traumatic disturbances as when a real-life mom fails to fulfill her archetypal stature.

The archetypes are the foundation of major mythologies, and correspond with gods, goddesses, and mythic heroes. They are found in the Major Arcana of the Tarot, may be seen and experienced through Kabbalistic path-working and shamanic trances, and are often met in dreams and projected onto real-life figures in times of crisis. One of the goals in every program of self-knowledge is to gain understanding of our particular interaction with them, and possibly to change those interactions from a childish to a more mature level.

The archetypes may be the 'gods,' each charged with particular responsibilities in the natural world.

Assiah. (Kabbalah—Tree of Life) The World of Action. The fourth and lowest of the Kabbalistic worlds corresponding to the material level, the world of sensation, the dominion of Primordial Earth and its four elements. Assiah is pictured either on the Tree of Life as Malkuth only, or as a fourth Tree of life below the other three.

Astral Body. The third body or level of consciousness, also called the Desire or Emotional Body. In the process of incarnation, the astral body is composed of the planetary energies in their aspects to one another to form a matrix for the physical body. This matrix is, in a sense, the true horoscope guiding the structure of the body and defining karmic factors.

The Astral Body is the Lower Self of Emotion, Imagination, Thinking, Memory, and Will—all the functions of the mind in response to sensory perception. It is the field of dreams and the subconscious mind. It is the vehicle for most psychic activities.

Yet, a distinction must be made: The Physical Body is the field of ordinary conscious mind and the Astral Body is that of the subconscious mind, and a doorway to the super conscious mind and the collective unconscious.

Astral Doorways. (Meditation) Meditation on certain objects may function (1) to induce an alternative state of consciousness, or (2) to bring access to certain areas of the subconscious and astral plane. Among the first are fascination devices that focus awareness and induce trance—crystal balls, magick mirrors, swinging pendulums, pools of ink, etc.—allowing the user to receive impressions. Among the second are Tarot Cards, Rune Symbols, I Ching Hexagrams, Egyptian Hieroglyphs, Hebrew Letters, Tattwas, and Yantras etc. used in meditation that open certain astral circuits and gain access to specific parts of the Astral Plane and to subjective states of consciousness.

Suggested Reading: Tyson: *Soul Flight, Astral Projection & the Magical Universe*

Astral Light. The 'substance' of the Astral Plane that responds to and records thought and feeling, forming memory.

Astral Plane. The second plane, sometimes called the Inner Plane or subjective world. It is an alternate dimension both coincident to our physical world and extending beyond it. Some believe it extends to other planets and allows for astral travel between them.

It is that level of concrete consciousness between the Physical/Etheric sphere of ordinary consciousness, and the Mental and Spiritual levels. It is where dreams, vision, and imagination are experienced and magical action shapes physical manifestation.

Astral Projection and Astral Travel. (Psychic Powers) It's desirable to treat these two subjects together because of the confusion in terminology over the years. Nonphysical movement in the familiar physical world is more likely to involve the Etheric body than the astral. The etheric is the energy double of the physical body, able to function separately from the physical body while connected to it with the 'silver cord' that transfers energy and consciousness between the two.

The etheric body can travel anywhere in the physical world, moving with the speed of thought, and can interact with the physical in a limited manner.

The astral body does not leave the physical body because it is not really an independent body, but is the subconscious mind and 'moves' within the field of consciousness without moving at all. Consciousness is everywhere, and in consciousness you can be anywhere. To the extent you want a body, you need to create a Body of Light in your imagination and then just imagine it doing what you want, going where you want.

But, the astral plane is not the physical world, and it lacks the 'solidity' of the physical plane, even though there is replication. However, things may appear on the astral that are not in the physical.

Suggested Reading: Bruce & Mercer: *Mastering Astral Projection* book and CD companion

—Denning and Phillips: *Practical Guide to Astral Projection, The Out-of-Body Experience*

—Goldberg: *Astral Voyages, Mastering the Art of Interdimensional Travel*

—Webster: *Astral Travel for Beginners, Transcend Time & Space with Out-of-Body Experiences*

Astral World. Just as we can speak of the physical plane and the physical world, so can we speak of the astral plane and the astral world. A "plane" (like a "level") is descriptive of the characteristics of the things that make up a world—the substance, energies, laws, etc. A "world," in contrast, is descriptive of how the things are put together, hence the landscape, the life-forms, the climates, and so forth.

The astral world has its own landscape, generally replicating the physical world, but is far more extensive, reaching wherever consciousness reaches. It has its own inhabitants, which include the astral bodies of the inhabitants of the physical world. Those astral inhabitants also include forms that have never incarnated into physical bodies, as well as temporary inhabitants created by humans through the power of imagination, emotion, and fantasy.

It is also possible that some creatures, like certain paranormal entities such as UFOs, Aliens, the Loch Ness and other 'monsters' that slip in and out of the physical world have their origin in the astral, and that mythical beings like dragons also exist in the lower astral close enough to the physical that they sometimes appear to the physical world inhabitants.

Astrology. (Astrology) While considered as an ancient form of divination, it is today used as a scientific approach to self-understanding and the forecasting of mundane (world-related) events: weather and climate changes, earth movements, economic and political events, and cultural trends. The horoscope provides a 'map' of planetary energies at any specific time and as projected at a particular location. That map is correlated with the meanings of those planetary energies as established through thousands of years of observation and the now established principles of horoscopic analysis and interpretation.

A horoscope calculated for the exact moment and place of birth a like a photograph taken of the complex relationship of planetary forces as reflected in the astral body. Since the astral is formative to the physical, this photograph tells the tale of the physical incarnation and of the Personality. Solar Return (birthday) horoscopes show the annual progression from the birth chart.

This scientific astrology has little to do with the simplistic 'birth sign' horoscopes found in popular media, which lump together approximately one-twelfth of the population as alike based purely on the position of the Sun in a particular zodiacal sign on their birthday. Thus, while there are some general similarities commonly shared by those of the same Sun Sign, there are nearly as often powerful planetary factors involved providing a substantial deviation from some of the generalities.

Suggested Reading: Llewellyn Publications: *The Daily Planetary Guide*, an annual guide to planetary positions and a beginner's guide to astrology

—Llewellyn: *Llewellyn's New A to Z Horoscope Maker and Interpreter,* A Comprehensive Self-Study Course

—Clement: *Mapping Your Birthchart, Understanding Your Needs & Potential* (with CD-ROM)

—Riske: *Llewellyn's Complete Book of Astrology, The Easy Way to Learn Astrology*

Attention. Focused awareness. Concentration. To "pay attention" is a conscious choice to limit perception and the work of consciousness to something specific.

Attraction. (Self-Empowerment) The principle involves believing yourself worthy and already in possession of those things you want. It functions best when used as a goal in our Self-Empowerment through Self-Hypnosis technique, which fully mobilizes your inner resources and leaves no doubt of your success.

Atziluth. (Kabbalah—Tree of Life) The first and highest Kabbalistic world, the divine world of the Archetypes. The domain of Primordial Fire. It corresponds to Kether, Chokmah, and Binah.

Aura. An egg-shaped sphere of energy extended as much as two to three feet beyond the physical body. It includes layers outward from the physical: the Etheric, Astral, Mental, and Spiritual bodies. The aura is known as the "magical mirror of the universe" in which our inner activities of thought and feeling are perceived in colors. It is also the matrix of planetary forces that shapes and sustains the physical body and the lower personality.

Clairvoyants may analyze the aura in relation to health, ethics, and spiritual development, and the aura can be shaped and its surface made to reflect psychic attacks back to their origin.

Suggested Reading: Andrews: *How to See and Read the Aura*

—Slate: *Aura Energy for Health, Healing & Balance*

—Webster: *Aura Reading for Beginners, Develop Your Psychic Awareness for Health & Success*

Autonomic nervous system. The 'lower intelligence' that safely runs the body functions without conscious awareness.

Awake. In contrast to being asleep, being awake supposedly says we are alert and perceptive to sensory input and the ongoing functions of ordinary consciousness. Nevertheless, self-observation will clearly show that there's more to being awake than having your eyes open! It's somewhat like having a dimmer on your light switch. Learn to turn up the intensity to become fully awake.

Awareness. Awareness is the focus of consciousness onto things, images, ideas, and sensations. Awareness is more than what we physically sense.

We do have psychic impressions independent of the physical apparatus. And we can focus our awareness on memories dredged up from the subconscious; we can focus on symbols and images and all the ideas, and memories, associated with them. We can turn our awareness to impressions from the astral and mental planes, and open ourselves to receiving information from other sources, from other planets, from other dimensions, and from other minds.

Awareness is how we use our consciousness. It is just as infinite as is consciousness, just as infinite as is the universe in all its dimensions and planes. When we speak of expanding or broadening our awareness, we are talking about paying attention to new impressions from new sources, and from other ways we can use our consciousness. Awareness is like the "Operating System" that filters incoming information, sometimes blocking "what we don't believe in."

Banishing. (Magick) A ritual approach to psychic self-protection. Many books provide the details of the practice, but a beginner should also gain understanding of the theory. The suggested title does that.

Become more than you are. (Self-Empowerment) You, we, all are a 'work-in-progress' towards fulfilling the potential of the whole person already existent as a 'matrix' of consciousness into which we are evolving. To "Become more than You are" is the goal of everyone who accepts the *opportunity* and *responsibility* of accelerated development and Self-Empowerment. It contrasts with the passive life that has no goals and accepts whatever is 'handed out.'

Suggested Reading: Regardie, with Chic and Sandra Tabatha Cicero: *The Tree of Life, An Illustrated Study in Magic*

Binah. (Kabbalah—Tree of Life) Aima Elohim, the Divine Mother, the third Sephirah on the Kabbalistic Tree of Life, Understanding. It is the primal feminine power. Also known as Ama, the dark sterile mother; Aima, the bright fertile mother; and Marah, the great sea. It is located at the top of the Pillar of Severity.

Name of God: Tetragrammaton Elohim
Archangel: Tzaphqiel (Contemplation of God)
Angelic Host: Aralim (Valiant Ones)
Astrological Correspondence: Saturn
Body: Right side of head
Colors: in Atziluth: crimson, in Briah: black, in Yetzirah:
    dark brown, in Assiah: gray flecked with pink
Consciousness: Neshamah, spiritual understanding

Element: Water
Magical Image: An old woman with long white hair
Symbols: All vaginal symbols
Tarot: The four Threes and four Queens

Body of Light. (Magick) Sometimes used as an alternative for the Astral Body, but more correctly as an image created ritually out of the astral light through the power of imagination and used by a magician as a vehicle for conscious perception and action.

Brain Waves. (Self-Hypnosis) The brain generates weak electrical impulses representative of its particular activities. As recorded by the electro-encephalograph (EEG), they fall into particular levels assigned Greek letters. Beta, at 14 to 26 cycles per second, is our normal waking state including focused attention, concentration, thinking, etc. Alpha, 8 to 13 cycles, is the next level down, characteristic of relaxation, alert receptivity, meditation, and access to the subconscious mind. It is at 8 cycles per second, the border between alpha and theta, that Trance occurs. Theta, 4 to 7, is lower yet and occurs just before (hypnopompic) or after (hypnagogic) sleep and is characteristic of light sleep, deep meditation, vivid imagery, and high levels of inner awareness. Delta, 0.5 to 3, is characteristic of deep sleep.

Brainstorming. Commonly a group search for new ideas, or for new applications for old ideas. It's best done as a rapid-fire, free-for-all, idea jam session opening the psychic faculties to inspiration.

Briah. (Kabbalah—Tree of Life) The second of the Kabbalistic four Worlds, the archangelic and creative world of pure intellect. The world of Creation and the dominion of Primordial Water. It corresponds to Chesed, Geburah, and Tiphareth on the Tree of Life.

Chakras. (Etheric Body) Psychic centers located in the aura functioning through the etheric body that exchange particular energies between the physical body and the personality, and the higher sources of energy associated with the planets, the Solar System, and the Cosmos.

There are seven traditional "master" chakras and dozens of minor ones located in such places as the palms of the hands, soles of the feet, joints of arms and legs, and just about any place traditionally adorned with jewelry.

Chakras are whirling centers of energy associated with particular areas of the body. In the Hindu tradition, *Muladhara* is located at the base of the spine and is the source of *Kundalini* and the power used in sex magic. *Svadisthana* is located at the sacrum. *Muladhara* and *Svadisthana* are linked to the physical body. *Manipura* is located at the solar plexus. *Muladhara,*

Svadisthana, and *Manipura* are together associated as the personality, and their energies can be projected through the solar plexus in such psychic phenomena as rapping, ectoplasm, and the creation of familiars. *Manipura* is linked to the lower astral body. *Anahata* is located at the heart and is associated with group consciousness. *Vishuddha* is located at the throat and is associated with clairvoyance. *Anahata* and *Ajna* are linked to the higher astral body. *Ajna* is located at the brow and is associated with clairvoyance. *Sahasrara* is located at the crown and is associated with spiritual consciousness. *Anahata, Vishuddha,* and *Sahasrara* are together associated as the spiritual self.

The master, or major, chakras are as follows. While we are listing some correspondences to planets, colors, and the Kabbalistic Sephiroth, there is considerable debate about these and the correlations cannot be specific because the chakras and the Sephiroth involve two different systems. Likewise, although not listed, there are differences between both these systems and those of Oriental martial arts and healing systems.

Muladhara, base of spine, color red, associated planet Saturn, Sephirah: Malkuth.

Svadisthana, genital area, color orange, associated planet Jupiter or Moon, Sephirah: Yesod.

Manipura, solar plexus below the navel, color yellow, associated planet Mars, Sephirah: none suggested.

Anahata, heart, color green, associated planet Sun or Venus, Sephirah: Tiphareth.

Vishuddha, throat, color blue, associated planet Mercury, Sephirah: Daath.

Ajna, brow, color indigo, associated planet Moon, Sephiroth: Chokmah and Binah.

Sahasrara, crown, color violet, associated planet none, Sephirah: Kether.

Suggested Reading: Judith: *Wheels of Life, A User's Guide to the Chakra System*

—Mumford: *Chakra & Kundalini Workbook, Psycho-spiritual Techniques for Health, Rejuvenation, Psychic Powers & Spiritual Rejuvenation*

Change. (Self-Empowerment) The purpose of this book is that of your Self-Empowerment. Instead of letting life happen to you, you can make life happen your way. But you have "to take charge" and "state your intentions."

Channeling. (Psychic Powers) Similar to, but not necessarily the same as, the spirit communication of mediumship. In both, however, one person serves as bridge between a spirit or spiritual intelligence and people of ordinary consciousness. In spirit communication, the medium is more often unaware of the communication; in channeling of spiritual intelligence, the channeler is more often aware and sometimes a participant.

Automatic Writing is a form of channeling in which a person, sometimes in trance, writes or even keyboards messages generally believed to originate with spiritual beings, or with aspects of the subconscious mind. The pendulum is likewise used as a communication device.

Chariot. (Tarot) The 7th Major Arcanum of the Tarot—image: a man on a chariot with two horses; Hebrew letter: Cheth; Divinatory meaning: victory, success; 18th path on the Tree of Life connecting Geburah to Binah.

Chesed. (Kabbalah—Tree of Life) The fourth Sephirah on the Tree of Life. It is also called Gedulah, Greatness. Located at the center of the Pillar of Mercy.
Name of God: El (God)
Archangel: Tzadkiel (Justice of God)
Angelic Host: Chashmalim (Shining Ones)
Astrological Correspondence: Jupiter
Body: Left shoulder
Colors: in Atziluth: deep violet, in Briah: blue, in Yetzirah:
    deep purple, in Assiah: deep azure flecked in yellow
Consciousness: Memory as part of Ruach, (the Conscious Self)
Element: Water
Magical Image: An old but mighty king on a throne
Tarot: The four Fours

Chiah. (Kabbalah—Tree of Life) Part of the soul located in Chokmah. It is Divine Will, the source of action.

Chokmah. (Kabbalah—Tree of Life) The second Sephirah on the Tree of Life, Wisdom. The primal masculine. Located at the top of the Pillar of Mercy.
Name of God: Yah (God)
Archangel: Raziel (Secret of God)
Angelic Host: Auphanim (Wheels)
Astrological Correspondence: The Zodiac, Sphere of the Stars
Body: Left side of head
Colors: in Atziluth: pure blue; in Briah: gray; in Yetzirah:
    iridescent pearl gray; in Assiah: white flecked with red, blue,
    and yellow.
Consciousness: Chiah, the spiritual will
Element: Fire

Human Soul: Chiah, the Divine Will
Magical Image: An old man
Symbols: All phallic symbols
Tarot: The four Twos and the four Kings

Circle. A temporary boundary within which a séance or magical operation may take place. The theory is that it becomes a kind of psychic container for the energies used in the operation and a barrier to unwanted energies from outside.

Clairaudience. (Psychic Powers) The psychic ability to hear things inaudible to most people, such as the voices of spirits, sometimes sounds of inanimate objects such as crystals, minerals, artifacts, etc.

Clairvoyance. (Psychic Powers) Sometimes called "ESP," the psychic ability to perceive things invisible to most people, such as auras, various health indicators, spirits, as well as events at a distance in space or time. It includes skrying (which see).

   Both clairaudience and clairvoyance, and other psychic skills, have been induced through hypnosis and self-hypnosis as well as developed through persistent exercises.

   Suggested Reading: Katz: *You Are Psychic, The Art of Clairvoyant Reading & Healing*

   —Owens: *Spiritualism & Clairvoyance for Beginners, Simple Techniques to Develop Your Psychic Abilities*

   —Slate and Weschcke: *Psychic Empowerment for Everyone*

Collective Unconscious. The memories of all of humanity, perhaps of more than human, and inclusive of the archetypes. The contents of the collective unconscious seem to progress from individual memories to universal memories as the person grows in his or her spiritual development and integration of the whole being. There is some suggestion that this progression also moves from individual memories through various groups or small collectives—family, tribe, race, and nation—so the character of each level is reflected in consciousness until the individual progresses to join in group consciousness with all humanity. This would seem to account for some of the variations of the universal archetypes each person encounters in life.

Conscious Mind. The 'middle' consciousness, the 'ordinary' consciousness, the 'objective' consciousness, the 'aware' consciousness with which we exercise control and direction over our 'awake' lives.

Consciousness. Everything that is, out of which Energy and Matter manifest and Life evolves. Consciousness is the beginning of all things and part of the trinity of Consciousness, Energy, and Matter. It includes all states of awareness and our experience of fear, love, hope, desire, happiness, sadness, depression, ecstasy, mystical union, etc. We experience connectedness through consciousness

"Consciousness just IS!" We can't really define consciousness because we are nothing but consciousness and consciousness cannot really define itself. "I AM THAT I AM." Consciousness is not a 'thing' nor is it a function of a 'thing' called the brain. Consciousness is expressed through the brain, but it exists outside the brain. Killing the brain doesn't kill consciousness but it limits its expression in the familiar physical world.

There are three "I" levels of consciousness:

I for Instinct, a function of the lower subconscious

I for Intelligence, a function of the ordinary consciousness

I for Intuition, a function of the super consciousness

Crystal Ball. A round ball of quartz crystal or glass used as focal point in skrying. Gazing at the ball, one enters into a trancelike state where dreamlike scenes and symbols are seen and interpreted. Similar aids are the Magic Mirror, a pool of black ink, or a piece of obsidian.

Suggested Reading: Andrews: *Crystal Balls & Crystal Bowls, Tools for Ancient Skrying & Modern Seership*

—Cunningham: *Divination for Beginners, Reading the Past, Present & Future*

Cyber Space. The 'new' Astral Plane. The role of the Internet as a search engine duplicates the memory resources of the Akashic Records; the instant transfer of communications via e-mail duplicate Mental Telepathy; the Social Networking tools duplicates the Astral Body as a kind of magic mirror; the role-playing Avatar duplicates the projected Body of Light. The expanding use of the Internet blends with similar functions on the Astral Plane to a degree that trains the user to function more directly, more *consciously,* in the subconscious mind and overcoming the barriers that previously existed.

Daath. (Kabbalah—Tree of Life) The "invisible" Sephirah on the Tree of Life, Knowledge. A passageway across the Abyss.

Astrological Correspondence: Sirius

Body: The Neck

Colors: in Atziluth: lavender; in Briah: pale silver gray; in Yetzirah: pure violet; in Assiah: gray flecked with gold

Consciousness: Ruach, the conscious self with Neshamah, the higher spiritual self

Element: Air
Symbols: The Empty Room, the Pyramid
Tarot: The Major Arcana

Death. (Tarot) The 13th Major Arcanum—image: Skeleton as the Grim Reaper; Hebrew letter: Nun; Divinatory meaning: change, transformation; 24th path on the Tree of Life connecting Netzach to Tiphareth.

Devil. (Tarot) The 15th Major Arcanum—image: usually a conventional-looking devil with horns and hooves standing on an altar to which are chained a man and a woman, alternatively the Pagan's Horned God; Hebrew letter: Ayin; Divinatory meaning: the instinctual drives of the subconscious mind; the 26th path on the Tree of Life connecting Hod to Tiphareth.

Divination. Prophesy and information by 'occult' methodologies.

1. By reading naturally produced signs ranging from the shape of clouds to the positions of planets (astrology).
2. By reading artificially produced signs ranging from tea leaves to the throwing of dice or dominoes.
3. By reading symbols such as the Tarot cards or the I Ching hexagrams.
4. By reading visions as seen in Dreams or in Trance.

   In each situation, something experienced is interpreted usually by means of long-established rules justified by many years of observation across many cultures. In most cases, these interpretations are supplemented by psychic factors of impressions or intuition naturally arising in either conscious or subconscious (trance) states. In expert situations, the divination is further complemented by contemporary knowledge of culture and subject so that the readings can have specific pertinence and application in contrast to esoteric vagueness.

Dream Interpretation. An important factor in Self-Empowerment is the more complete utilization of lines of communication between levels of consciousness. While commercial "dream dictionaries" rarely have much value, one that you compile yourself may be immensely helpful. Through the regular use of a Dream Journal, you become familiar with your own symbol meanings and can explore each further for more insight. When you actually pay attention to your dreams, they start to pay attention to you and can deliver information and even guidance of immediate application.

Dreaming True. Programmed dreaming where a question or an intention is formulated before sleep, and left to the subconscious mind to respond with an answer or an action. It can also be effectively programmed with self-hypnosis. It generally requires an extensive and current knowledge of the subjects of which questions are asked. Thus, if you want to know the winner in a forthcoming horse race, you need to know the names of the horses running, background information on the horses and their jockeys, their owners, and other information that may be presented in symbolic code by the subconscious mind in the dream state.

Dreams. Stories experienced during sleep. Some dreams seem merely to be translations of physical experiences, while others are presented with the drama and richness of cinema, and others seem to be ways we assimilate new information. Dreams are also a function of the subconscious mind and deliberate dreaming is a doorway into the subconscious and its connection to the collective unconscious. Much of the power of dreams relates to the ways in which archetypes are involved in them.

Suggested Reading: Gonzalez-Wippler: *Dreams & What They Mean to You*

—Gongloff: *Dream Exploration, A New Approach*

Egregor. (Magick) An artificial entity created of astral light by magical intent or religious devotion, often in the form of a guardian creature (such as an Eagle or Lion) to protect a building or a spiritual group. The form can originate in mythology or be adapted from folklore and can be ritually charged with additional functions such as observing distant events, carrying out an act of revenge, or to serve as a focus of devotion to unite the group.

Elemental. (1) Nonhuman nature spirits associated with the state, quality, and character of the five elements or Tattwas.

Air (gaseous; mediating, embracing, and pervasive; intellect): Sylphs

Earth (solid; stable and enduring; sensation): Gnomes

Fire (energy; active, energizing, and transforming; will):
Salamanders

Spirit, Ether (underlying; universal and originating; awareness): Spirits

Water (fluid; receptive and responsive; feeling): Undines

(2) A thought form charged with energy and intention by a magician to carry out a particular operation, such as a household guardian.

Emotion. "Energy in motion." Emotion is a dynamic and powerful response to something perceived that connects to universal human experience and archetypes. Emotion is the energy 'powering' most intentional psychic and magical operations, the energy responsible for many types of psychic phenomena, possibly including hauntings, poltergeists, rapping, etc. where there is potential for the emotion to have been 'recorded' in the woodwork of the building. Emotion is found in Netzach as part of Ruach, the Conscious Self.

Emperor. (Tarot) The 4th Major Arcanum—image: Crowned and enthroned man; Hebrew letter: Heh; Divinatory meaning: power, authority, fatherhood; 15th path on the Tree of Life connecting Tiphareth to Chokmah.

Empress. (Tarot) The 3rd Major Arcanum—image: Crowned and enthroned woman, usually pregnant; Hebrew letter: Daleth; Divinatory meaning: fertility, productivity, fulfillment, motherhood; 14th path on the Tree of Life connecting Binah to Chokmah.

"End of the world as we know it." A phrase based on the Mayan Prophecy, that the world "as we know it" will end on December 21, 2012, that there will be a dramatic rebirth of the human spirit and a new global civilization structured to meet the challenges of international terrorism starting in 2001, religious extremism, the financial collapse of 2008, cultural degradation, and other common threats to planetary survival.

New planetary-sized institutions and international standards will likely be required of nations to participate in new economic, security, educational, legal, health, etc. organizations.

ESP. (Psychic Powers) See Extrasensory Perception.

Ether. Identical with the Hindu *Akasha* and the fifth element in Western Magic, Spirit that is believed to originate the other four: Earth, Water, Fire, and Air. Also called Astral Light, Ch'i, Odic Force, Orgone, Prana, Vril, the Force. It can be concentrated and directed by will, and intensified by breath.

Etheric Body. (Etheric Body) The second, or energy body that is closest to the physical body. As with all the subtle bodies, it has two layers:

The first, sometimes called the "Etheric Double," is fully coincident with the physical body in health and extends about an inch beyond physical skin. It is the psycho-physical circuitry of the human body (the chakras, nadis, and meridians) through which the life-force flows under direction of the astral matrix. To clairvoyant vision, it is the health aura and appears as very fine needles of radiation—standing straight up in health and lying down in illness.

The second layer, along with the astral and mental bodies, forms the egg-shaped aura surrounding the human body. It is an interface between the individual and dynamic planetary energies and cosmic forces that sustain life.

Etheric Plane. The Energy Plane between the Physical and Astral planes. Its energies are in constant movement, like tides and currents, ruled by the Moon, Sun, and Planets and moving in cycles.

Etheric Projection. (Etheric Body) A portion of the etheric body, sometimes along with other etheric material for added substance, can be formed as a vehicle for the operator's consciousness and projected to other physical locations. Being of near physical substance and energy, it is sensitive to certain physical materials, like iron and silver. It can be injured, and such injuries will repercuss back to the physical body.

The etheric body can also be shaped to resemble other entities, and is a factor in the lore of were-wolves and were-leopards.

Etheric Revenant. (Etheric Body) This is the foundation for vampire lore. As with the ancient Egyptian practice of mummification, the preserved body—hidden and protected from disturbance including the effect of sunlight—provides a base for the continued use of the etheric body by the personality of a deceased person. The etheric body has to be nourished with substances rich with life energy, like blood.

Expectancy Effect. The effect of expectation on the future, to include personal performance and outcomes, with expectations of success typically facilitating success.

Extrasensory Perception (ESP). (Psychic Powers) The awareness of, or response to, events, conditions, and situations independently of known sensory mechanisms or processes. You can develop your extrasensory perception (ESP) powers that include telepathy or the ability to communicate mentally with others, precognition or the ability to perceive future events, and clairvoyance or the ability to mentally perceive conditions and distant events. You can develop your PK powers or your ability to mentally influence happenings and processes.

Fascination devices. (Self-Hypnosis) Crystal balls (often made of glass), crystals, cut glass, mirrors, magick mirrors (black glass), swinging pendants, crystal bowls, painted eyes, icons and images painted in flashing colors (complimentary colors placed together), spinning disks, and other devices that focus the attention but tire the vision. Sometimes a small focal object is placed above the eye level forcing one to soon close the eyes. Combined with either a hetero or an internal dialogue, their use can be very effective in hypnotic induction.

Suggested Reading: Andrews: *Crystal Balls & Crystal Bowls, Tools for Ancient Skrying & Modern Seership*

—Cunningham: *Divination for Beginners, Reading the Past, Present & Future*

Field. The First Thing, the field of manifestation. Consciousness, from which first Energy and then Matter arose as Energy/Matter packets that manifest as Waves or Particles. The Field is the Source for all that follows—today as yesterday and as tomorrow. The Field can be accessed through deliberate thought and responds to emotion expressed with intention. Through the Field we can change 'reality,' hence it is the field of magic, phenomena, and of miraculous things that matter.

Suggested Reading: McTaggart: *The Field, the Quest for the Secret Force of the Universe*

—McTaggart: *The Intention Experiment, Using Your Thoughts to Change Your Life and the World*

Focusing tools. (Self-Hypnosis) Like Fascination Devices, these aid by attracting either the visual or the auditory senses and are used to calm the mind during induction.

Fool. (Tarot) Generally numbered "0" or 22nd of the Major Arcana—image: variously a Court Jester and a dog about to step off a cliff, a naked child with a dog, a pilgrim in a strange land, or an enthused rider with his dog jumping his horse across the chasm between the worlds; Hebrew letter: Aleph, Divinatory meaning: fool-hardy courage, determination, act of faith; 11th path on the Tree of Life connecting Chokmah to Kether.

Forgotten Memories. (Self-Hypnosis) Memories are retained in the subconscious and may be recalled using various techniques including word association, asking questions, dialogue, and 'sleeping on it.' Nothing is truly forgotten, but things may have been insignificant at the time, painful and so repressed, overshadowed by larger events, etc. Memories can be recovered if you know what you are looking for and if you know they are pertinent. Sometimes, events will remind you and otherwise tell you that something significant is missing.

Four Divisions of Soul. (Kabbalah—Tree of Life) As pictured on the Tree of Life, these levels are:
1. Neshamah, which is itself divided into three parts:
   a. Yechidah (the superego), centered in Kether, is our Divine Self
   b. Chiah, centered in Chokmah, is our True Will
   c. Neshamah, centered in Binah, is our Intuition
2. Ruach (the ego), consisting of Chesed, Geburah, Tiphareth, Netzach, and Hod, is our Mind
3. Nephesch (lower self), centered in Yesod, is our subconsciousness

4. Guph. The lowest part of the soul, centered in Malkuth. A low level of subconscious intelligence allied to the physical body. The autonomic nervous system.

Four Worlds. (Kabbalah—Tree of Life) The four fundamental levels of being or consciousness as considered in the Kabbalah:

1. Atziluth (nearness): the archetypal or divine world—Fire and the Spiritual Plane
2. Briah (creation): the archangelic world of eternal patterns of Platonic ideas—Water and the Mental Plane
3. Yetzirah (formation): the angelic world of force and form—Air and the Astral Plane
4. Assiah (action): the physical world of matter and energy—Earth and the Physical Plane

In relation to the Tree of Life, the Four Worlds are presented in two different ways

A. Four different levels on one Tree:
   a. Atziluth corresponds to the first through third Sephiroth: Kether, Chokmah and Binah
   b. Briah corresponds to the fourth through sixth Sephiroth: Chesed, Geburah and Tiphareth
   c. Yetzirah corresponds to the seventh through ninth Sephiroth: Netzach, Hod and Yesod
   d. Assiah corresponds to the tenth Sephirah: Malkuth

B. Four different Trees one on top of the other so that Malkuth of the highest Tree is also Kether of the next Tree lower, and so on

Meditation on both these ways will be meaningful.

Geburah. (Kabbalah—Tree of Life) Harsh judgment, the fifth Sephirah on the Kabbalistic Tree of life, Severity. It is the potential for evil. It is located in the center of the Pillar of Severity.

Name of God: Elohim Gibor (Almighty God)

Archangel: Kamael (He who sees God)

Angelic Host: Seraphim (Fiery Serpents)

Astrological Correspondence: Mars

Body: Left shoulder

Colors: in Atziluth: orange, in Briah: red, in Yetzirah: bright scarlet, in Assiah: red flecked with black

Consciousness: The Will as part of Ruach (the Conscious Self)

Element: Fire

Magical Image: A warrior king (or queen), fully armored, standing in a chariot

Symbol: The pentagram

Tarot: The four Fives

Gedulah. (Kabbalah—Tree of Life) An alternative name for Chesed, meaning Greatness.

Global Civilization. The belief that humanity in the twentieth century struggled to create the first global civilization based on a commonality of Hollywood-centered entertainment, international political organizations growing out of World War II and the Cold War, the European Union, a world economy, a common currency, universal education, universal human law, and free trade.

An essential role has depended on the decline in religious conflict so that religions are no longer being so divisive, along with a growing acceptance of nonsectarian spirituality.

Great Plan, the. Some occultists believe that there is a Plan guiding the evolution of human consciousness to its eventual reunion with the ultimate Source.

Suggested Reading: Any of the books by Alice Bailey

Great Work. The path of self-directed spiritual growth and development.

Group Mind. The collective consciousness of a group or team of people working together with their thoughts and feelings focused on the same projects or studies. It may be a spontaneous function of a group of like-mined people or deliberately created by a magical group or a functional organization such as a business corporation or working partnership. It was part of the teachings of Napoleon Hill, author of *Think and Grow Rich.*

Group Soul. The collective consciousness of a community, herd, nation, ethnic group, or nation, reflecting and then reinforcing distinctive behavior, thoughts, and culture.

Guided Imagery. (Meditation) The use of suggestion and visualization to guide thought processes, typically to promote a positive state of physical relaxation and personal well being. Guided imagery can, however, be used to induce a trance state or as a goal-oriented technique for managing stress or pain, overcoming fear, breaking unwanted habits, slowing aging, and promoting wellness, to mention but a few of the possibilities.

Guided Meditation. (Meditation) A meditation led by an experienced guide following established inner pathways to access particular iconic collections of knowledge and experience. A typical example would be found in

Kabbalistic Path-Workings progressing on the Path from one Sphere to another on the Tree of Life.

Suggested Reading: Lorenzo-Fuentes: *Meditation*

—Clayton: *Transformative Meditation, Personal & Group Practice to Access Realms of Consciousness*

Guph. (Kabbalah—Tree of Life) The lowest part of the soul, centered in Malkuth. A low level of subconscious intelligence allied to the physical body. The autonomic nervous system.

Hanged Man. (Tarot) The 12th Major Arcanum—image: Man hanging by one foot with the other crossed behind; Hebrew letter: Mem; Divinatory meaning: suspension, delay, reversal, personal sacrifice; 23rd path on the Tree of Life connecting Hod to Geburah.

Healing through Self-Hypnosis. (Self-Hypnosis) Based on the premise that a supreme healing force exists in everyone, healing through Self-Hypnosis accesses that force and focuses in on specific goals related to healing, both mental and physical. This concept also recognizes the existence of healing dimensions beyond the self and our capacity through Self-Hypnosis to tap into them.

Health Diagnosis through Self-Hypnosis. (Self-Hypnosis) This concept is based on the premise that you alone know yourself best. Through Self-Hypnosis, you can not only identify the conditions relevant to your health, you can intervene directly in ways that promote healing. Various techniques are employed, but the most common includes a visual (inner) survey of the body itself with the expectation that the subconscious mind will seize the opportunity to call attention to areas of the body with need for medical intervention.

Hermit. (Tarot) The 9th Major Arcanum—image: an old man in a hooded robe with staff and lantern standing in a circle, and accompanied by a serpent; Hebrew letter: Yod; Divinatory meaning: Wisdom, Secret Knowledge, Solitary Practice; 20th path on the Tree of Life connecting Tiphareth to Chesed.

Hexagram. (1) A six-pointed star consisting of two superimposed triangles, one whose apex is up and the other apex down. The upward triangle is masculine, the downward is feminine—together they symbolize union of energies or sexual congress. In ritual magic, they are used to invoke or to banish planetary forces. (2) One of sixty-four combinations of long and broken lines used in the I Ching (or Yi King) system of Chinese divination that are traditionally determined by throwing Yarrow Sticks, or by means of coins (heads, tails), dice, dominoes, or other means. (3) As a symbol, it is the Hebrew "Star of David."

> Suggested Reading: Regardie, with the Ciceros: *The Tree of Life, An Illustrated Study in Magic*
>
> —Kraig: *Modern Magick, Eleven Lessons in the High Magickal Arts*
>
> —McElroy: *I Ching for Beginners, A Modern Interpretation of the Ancient Oracle*
>
> —Nishavdo: *I Ching of Love*—a boxed set of 64 illustrated cards with booklet

Hierophant. (Tarot) The 5th Major Arcanum—image: Pope or other major religious leader; Hebrew letter: Vau; Divinatory meaning: Authority, Wisdom, Spirituality; 16th path on the Tree of Life connecting Yesod to Tiphareth.

High Priestess. (Tarot) The 2nd Major Arcanum—image: a high priestess seated in front of a veil, crescent moon at her feet with the horns upward; Hebrew letter: Gimel; Divinatory meaning: Intuition, Revealed Wisdom, Ebb and Flow; 13th path on the Tree of Life connecting Tiphareth to Kether.

Higher Planes. (1) A general reference to levels above the physical—generally meaning Etheric, Astral, Mental, and Spiritual. (2) A reference to levels above that being discussed, and generally meaning planes above the Spiritual or that are commonly grouped into the Spiritual Plane. Planes refer to (a) levels of manifestation and (b) levels of the whole person—as 'bodies.'

Higher Self. The super conscious mind in Tiphareth that mediates between the Divine Self and the Lower Personality. Historically it has been suppressed through the denial of knowledge about self and the potentials of the whole person. The Higher Self appears in dreams and in visions as a Guide to the Lower Self.

Hod. (Kabbalah—Tree of Life) The eighth Sephirah on the Tree of Life, Splendor. Located at the base of the Pillar of Form and Severity.
Name of God: Elohim Tzaboath (God of Armies)
Archangel: Raphael (Healing of God)
Angelic Host: Beni Elohim (Children of the Gods)
Astrological Correspondence: Mercury
Body: Left hip
Colors: in Atziluth: violet purple, in Briah: orange, in Yetzirah:
 reddish russet, in Assiah: yellowish brown flecked with white
Consciousness: The Intellect as part of Ruach (the Conscious Self)
Element: Water

Magical Image: a warrior hermaphrodite
Symbol: The caduceus
Tarot: The four Eights

Holy Guardian Angel. (Magick) The Divine Self that can be contacted by the lower self through spiritual and magical practices. But, that contact has to be "earned" through the efforts and development of the lower self.

Horoscope. (Astrology) A 'map' of the planetary positions at any moment of time as seen for a point on the earth's surface. It is the form from which astrological interpretations are given based upon thousands of years of observed coincidental phenomena.

Suggested Reading: Perry: *Saturn Cycles, Mapping Changes in Your Life*

—Clement: *Mapping Your Birthchart, Understanding Your Needs & Potential*

Hypnosis (see also Self-Hypnosis). An Altered State of Conscious that provides a bridge to the subconscious mind by which conscious suggestions mobilize subconscious resources including current and past-life memories, and exercise certain control over physical body responses to external stimuli and internal functions, access areas of the collective unconscious, and channel communication between astral and mental levels and the physical level. The hypnotic trance has been associated with various psychic abilities.

As the historical and scientific advancements in hypnosis continue, interest in hypnosis has slowly expanded to include self-hypnosis and its applications, particularly toward *self -development and personal empowerment.* That trend is due in large part to the recognition that hypnosis, to be effective, depends not only on the skill of the hypnotist, but even more importantly, on the receptivity of the participant. That recognition places the participant, rather than the hypnotist, at the center of the induction process. The result is a moving away from an authoritative, often dramatic induction approach that *commanded* the participant to respond toward a more permissive, person-centered approach that *permitted* the participant to respond. That change is based on the premise that *hypnotic suggestions become effective only when accepted and integrated by the cooperative participant._*

Suggested Reading: Hewitt: *Hypnosis for Beginners, Reach New Levels of Awareness & Achievement*

Hypnotic Induction. (Self-Hypnosis) The procedures preliminary to the actual hypnosis session, starting with relaxation of the body and calmness of mind, focus on the established intention of the session, and the development of a concise statement of that intention as accomplished.

I AM. (Self-Hypnosis) This phrase invokes the higher self in a powerful self-affirmation used in self-hypnosis in a goal statement setting forth the desired condition as now present.

I Ching. A Chinese divinatory system of 64 'hexagrams' that express the dynamic flow of energies into their physical manifestation. Like most divination, it is a manipulative system calling forth the practitioner's psychic abilities.

> Suggested Reading: McElroy: *I Ching for Beginners, A Modern Interpretation of the Ancient Oracle*
> —Brennan: *The Magical I Ching*

Icons. It is through symbols and images, and icons, that we open the doors of our inner perception. The great secrets of magicians, shamans, and modern scientists are in the associations they attach to such icons, and in the power of certain signs and formulae to function as circuits and pathways—not in the brain but in consciousness.

Images. (Self-Empowerment) It is through symbols and images, and icons, that we open the doors of our inner perception. The great secrets of magicians, shamans, and modern scientists are in the associations they attach to such icons, and in the power of certain signs and formulae to function as circuits and pathways—not in the brain but in consciousness.

Imagination. The ability to form and visualize images and ideas in the mind, especially of things never seen or experienced directly. The imagination is an amazing and powerful part of our consciousness because it empowers our creativity—the actual ability to create. Imagination is found in Tiphareth as part of Ruach, the Conscious Self.

Induction. See Hypnotic Induction.

Inner-Directed Aquarian Man. (Self-Empowerment) The Inner-Directed person holds independent views derived through rational study and/or intuitive processes in contrast to the outer-directed person who 'follows the crowd' or accepts the guidance of authority figures without reasonable questions. 'Inner-Directed' has also been associated with the Aquarian Age individual man in contrast to the Piscean Age with its symbolism of fish that swim in groups. The outer-directed person is perceived as easily manipulated because of his dependence on outer authority.

Inner Divinity. (Self-Empowerment) The belief that each person has a 'Divine Spark' or part of the Divine Creator at his core. As the person evolves and grows in wholeness, he becomes more and more closely identified with his Divinity until an ultimate unity is accomplished.

Interactive Relaxation. Inducing physical relaxation through intervention into the mental functions related to relaxation. Common examples are the use of visualization and suggestion to induce a peaceful, relaxed state.

Intelligence. (1) The rational and cognitive powers of mind. Intelligence is found in Hod as part of Ruach, the Conscious Self. (2) An independent, nonhuman entity capable of communication across space or dimension.

International Parapsychology Research Foundation (IPRF). Established at Athens State University in 1970 by Joe H. Slate, Ph.D., this foundation is committed to the study of parapsychology and related topics. It has conducted extensive research and established student scholarships in perpetuity at Athens State University and the University of Alabama. The president of the foundation is District Judge Sam Masdon of Montgomery, AL. For more information, contact Joe H. Slate, Ph.D. at joehslate@aol.com

Interdimensional Interaction Program. Nothing more clearly illustrates our spiritual essence than our capacity to interact with the spirit dimension. Our awareness of spirit guides and, in some instances, the departed, illustrates our capacity as spiritual beings to interact with the spiritual realm. To explore that interaction and its empowering potentials, the Interdimensional Interaction Program was formed at Athens State University under the auspices of the Foundation. A major objective of the program was to determine the relevance of self-hypnosis to spirituality, to include mediumistic communications.

Intuition. A blinding flash of insight answering a question or solving a problem originating at the Soul level of consciousness.

Judgement. (Tarot) Also spelled 'Judgment.' The 20th Major Arcanum— image: resurrection day with an angel blowing a trumpet as the dead arise from their graves; Hebrew letter: Shin; Divinatory meaning: renewal, rebirth, the final outcome; the 31st path on the Tree of Life connecting Malkuth to Hod.

Jungian Psychology. Also called Analytic Psychology—the system developed by C. G. Jung. After studying with Freud, he advanced a more spiritual approach to psychotherapy evolving out of his studies of occult traditions and practices including, in particular, alchemy, astrology, dream interpretation, the I Ching, the Tarot, and spiritualism.

For Jung, the whole range of occult and religious phenomena evolved out of the relationship between the individual consciousness and the collective unconscious. While the personal unconscious or subconscious mind is the 'lower' part of the individual consciousness, it is through it that we also experience and have experience of the elements of the collective unconscious—most importantly the role of the archetypes.

The archetypes are 'collectives' of images and energies relating to (1) role-specific functional, formative, and universal experiences such as Mother, Father, Lover, Judge, Hero, etc.; (2) those that are more personal with karmic content including the Shadow (repressions), the Anima (expressions of the Feminine in men), the Animus (expressions of the Masculine in women); and (3) the Self (the evolving whole person that overshadows the personality).

Justice. (Tarot) The 8th Major Arcanum—image: a woman with a sword in one hand and the scales of justice in the other; Hebrew letter: Lamed; Divinatory meaning: legal matters, balance; the 22nd path on the Tree of Life connecting Tiphareth to Geburah.

Kabbalah. A complete system of knowledge about all the dimensions of the universe and of the human psyche organized into 'the Tree of Life' diagram showing the inner construction and the connections between levels and forms of consciousness, energy, and matter. It provides a resource for understanding and applying the principles of Magick, for understanding the dynamics of the psyche, and for interpreting human history and action. The present day Tarot specifically relates to the Tree of Life.

"The Universe began not with an atom or a subatomic particle, but with a thought in the mind of God. This thought of Creation encompassed a world in which every human being would enjoy happiness and fulfillment, free from any form of chaos or pain. This is what the Creator desires and intends.

"But bringing about the realization of the Creator's desire is up to us. For the manifestation of complex fulfillment to take place, we need to evolve into our truest, greatest selves. In our thoughts, our feelings, and our actions, we need to erase negativity and replace darkness with Light. It is for this purpose that the teachings and tools of Kabbalah were given to all humanity."

By Rav Berg in the Introduction, *The Sacred Zohar*, 2007, The Kabbalah Center, Los Angeles, 2007.

Suggested Reading: Stavish: *Kabbalah for Health and Wellness*

—Regardie and Cicero: *The Middle Pillar, the Balance Between Mind & Magic*

Kether. (Kabbalah—Tree of Life) The first Sephirah on the Tree of Life, Crown. It is located at the top of the Middle Pillar.

God Name: Eheieh (I AM)

Archangels: Metatron (The Prince of Countenances)

Angelic Host: Chaioth ha-Qodesh (Holy Living Creatures)

Astrological Correspondence: Primum Mobile (the turning movement in Space)

Body: Above the crown of the head

Colors: in Atziluth: pure brilliance, in Briah: brilliant white, in Yetzirah: brilliant white, in Assiah: white flecked with gold.

Consciousness: The Yechidah, Divine Self

Element: Air

Magical Image: A human face looking right

Symbol: The point

Tarot: The four Aces

"Know Thyself." This motto was inscribed on the sixth-century BCE temple of Apollo at Delphi and quoted by several ancient writers, some of whom attributed it to Solon. It has been since quoted by thousands if not millions of self-help, motivational, and spiritual writers and teachers.

Kundalini. (Etheric Body) The Life Force rising from the base of the spine, the *Muladhara* chakra, and animating the body, our sexuality, the etheric body, and passing through the chakras to join with its opposite force descending through the *Sahasrara* chakra to open our higher consciousness.

Suggested Reading: Mumford: *A Chakra & Kundalini Workbook, Psycho-Spiritual Techniques for Health, Rejuvenation, Psychic Powers & Spiritual Realization*

—Paulson: *Kundalini and the Chakras, Evolution in this Lifetime – A Practical Guide*

Life Between Lives. Following the belief in reincarnation, there is a period between the previous life and the next life during which the past life is reviewed and the next life planned.

Suggested Reading: Newton: *Destiny of Souls, New Case Studies of Life Between Lives*

—Newton: *Journey of Souls, Case Studies of Life Between Lives*

—Newton: *Life Between Lives, Hypnotherapy for Spiritual Regression*

Life Journey. The 'journey' through life that each person makes. It is the 'story' of one single lifetime.

Life's Purpose. (Self-Empowerment) We are here to grow, to become more than we are. Each of us has the ability to apply our inherent powers and our emerging skills to the challenge of accelerating personal growth.

Loading. (Self-Hypnosis) Associating an I AM sentence and a symbol with a full description and image of that which is desired. Then the sentence and symbol are vehicles for the entire operation and are used in self-hypnosis to convey the desired goal to the subconscious.

Lovers. (Tarot) The 6th Major Arcanum—image: a young couple (with a serpent present) blessed by an angel, or the chained maiden rescued by the hero; Hebrew letter: Zayin; Divinatory meaning: release, inspiration, new start; the 17th path on the Tree of Life connecting Tiphareth to Binah.

Lower Self. The conscious mind and the subconscious mind, together, are the Lower Self.

Magic. (Magick) The power to change things in conformity with will or desire. It is a function of focused consciousness accompanied by a force of Love intending change by reaching down into the Universal Field where everything exists as potential until affected by the operation of magic. This means that magic is happening all the time, but as magicians we have the opportunity and responsibility as co-creators to direct change in accordance with personal desire or what is called 'The Great Plan,' meaning no more and no less than whatever the underlying purpose of creation is.

As "low (or practical) magic," it is the intentional ritual action—supported by various physical correspondences with particular herbs, astrological factors, symbols, etc. lending strength to the visualized accomplishment through psychic powers—to make things happen as a materialization of desire.

As "High Magick," it is the intentional ceremonial action—supported by particular philosophical correspondences—to bring about self-development, including increased psychic skills, to the realization of the whole person, which is what the Great Plan is all about.

Magic Mirror. (Self-Hypnosis) A device, similar to the crystal ball, to focus attention in a process of self-hypnosis to open a channel between the conscious mind and the astral world, i.e., the subconscious mind.

Magical Personality. (Magick) It is a constructed personality, given a magical name, that can be compared to the created Avatar in cyber games. It is an idealized self-image for the whole person you are coming to be.

Magician. (Tarot) The first Major Arcanum—image: a magician standing behind his altar upon which there are various magical tools; Hebrew letter: Beth; Divinatory meaning: will, intelligence, communication, skill; the 12th path of the Tree of Life Binah to Kether.

Malkuth. (Kabbalah—Tree of Life) The tenth Sephirah on the Tree of Life, the Kingdom. It is located at the bottom of the Middle Pillar.
God Name: Adonai (Lord)
Archangels: Metatron and Sandalphon
Angelic Host: Ishim (Humanity)
Astrological Correspondence: The Elements
Body: The feet
Colors: in Atziluth: clear yellow, in Briah: citrine, olive, russet and
    black, in Yetzirah: citrine, olive, russet, and black flecked with
    gold, in Assiah: black rayed with yellow.
Consciousness: Guph, the physical body
Element: Earth
Magical Image: A young woman sitting on a throne
Symbol: An altar or temple
Tarot: The four Tens, the four Pages (or Princesses)

Manipura. (Etheric Body) Chakra located at the solar plexus below the navel, color yellow, associated planet Mars, associated Sephirah: none suggested.

Mantra. (Meditation) A word or phrase, usually in Sanskrit, Hebrew, or Latin, repeated or chanted repeatedly as a way to still the mind in meditation, and/or to instill a particular feeling or to invoke a special state of consciousness.

Matrix. (Etheric Body) The background framework for all and any manifestation. It is a union of Consciousness in the Universal Field of primary energy/matter potentials. The universal matrix is the pattern for evolving universe and all within it. The individual matrix is the pattern of energy/matter guiding the development and function of each life-form. It is mostly a function of Mental, Astral, and Etheric levels of consciousness guided by an intention expressed at the Soul level. It functions as the Etheric Body.
    Suggested Reading: Bradden: *The Divine Matrix, Bridging Time, Space, Miracles, and Belief*

Mayan Prophecy for 2012. A prediction that the world (at least as we know it) will end on December 21, 2012.

Meaning to Life. (Self-Empowerment) One of the most challenging questions any of us will ever confront. We can say that our Life's Purpose is 'to grow, to become more than we are,' but purpose and meaning may not be exactly the same thing. 'Meaning' may be either personal or for all of us—either way, it is probably best discovered for oneself. Meditate on it often.

Meditation. (Meditation) (1) An emptying of the mind of all thoughts and 'chatter,' often by concentrating only on the slow inhalation and exhalation of breath, and is characterized by slow alpha and theta waves. It induces relaxation and a 'clean slate' preparatory to receiving psychic impressions. (2) A careful thinking about a particular subject in a manner that brings access to physical memories as well as astral and mental level associations of knowledge about that subject. (3) A state of consciousness characterized by relaxed alertness reducing sensory impressions with increased receptivity to inner plane communications.

Suggested Reading: Clement: *Meditation for Beginners, Techniques for Awareness, Mindfulness & Relaxation*

—Paulson: *Meditation as Spiritual Practice*

Medium. (Psychic Powers) See also "Channel." Most mediums enter a trance state and then—often through the agency of a "control" or "guide," enable communication with a discarnate person. Often the Control speaks for the Spirit seeking communication.

Suggested Reading: Mathews: *Never Say Goodbye, A Medium's Stories of Connecting with Your Loved Ones*

Mediumship. (Psychic Powers) The study and development of the skill necessary to function as a spiritual medium facilitating communication between the worlds of spirit and the living. See also Spiritualism.

Suggesting Reading: Eynden: *So You Want to be a Medium? A Down-to-Earth Guide*

Memory. Memory is found in Chesed as part of Ruach, the Conscious Self.

Memory Palace. An imagined palace in which you learn to visualize rooms in a carefully designed pattern and then you associate learned facts and lessons with similar facts and lessons in assigned rooms.

Mental Body. The fourth body. The mental body "thinks" in abstract rather than emotional form. The lower mental body unites with the astral and etheric bodies as the personality for current incarnation. The higher mental body is home to the Soul between incarnations.

Mental Plane. The third plane up from the physical/etheric between the Astral and the Spiritual Planes. It is the plane of abstract consciousness, where we find meaning, patterns, the laws of nature and mathematics, number. and form. It is the plane where all thought is shared. It is the upper home for the Akashic Records shared with the astral.

Mental Telepathy. (Psychic Powers) Mind-to-mind communication by non-physical means. Usually, an image of the intended receiver is held in mind while a simple message, such as "Call me," is projected. Once the message is sent, it is important to "let go" of it rather than doing constant repetition.

Mesmerism. Modern science first became involved in hypnosis with the work of the Austrian physician Franz Anton Mesmer (1734–1815). Mesmer developed a theory called 'animal magnetism' using magnets as healing tools to influence what was believed to be a magnetic field surrounding the physical body. The practice, which became known as mesmerism, included passing a magnet (or at times a twig of wood) over a wound to stop bleeding resulting from bloodletting. An investigation conducted by a French Board of Inquiry, which included the American Benjamin Franklin, concluded that the purported effects of magnets were instead the consequences of the subject's imagination. Franklin's research team further concluded that *the healings were due to the patient's own powers*, not those of the magnet. That finding was to become a major step toward the recognition of hypnosis as a scientific approach with potential for self-development and desired change (Ellenberger 1980).

Middle Pillar Exercise. (Self-Empowerment) A very powerful and effective daily ritual/exercise for activating the five psychic centers of the Middle Pillar in the body. In ways, it resembles the arousing of chakras, but follows the Kabbalistic pattern, and the concept of Light descending and then circulating. Each center is visualized as a sphere of colored light about six inches across one at a time, and then its God Name vibrated four times. After all five centers are established, currents of energy are visualized rising internally from the base and then descending externally to enter again to energize the aura.

The exercise is preceded by the Kabbalistic Cross and the Lesser Banishing Ritual of the Pentagram in the following complete sequence.

Kabbalistic Cross. Standing, feet together, facing east, and using the right hand:

1. Touch the forehead and say/vibrate ATOH (Thou Art)
2. Bring the hand down to the groin area and say/vibrate MALKUTH (the Kingdom)
3. Touch the right shoulder, and say/vibrate VE-GEBURAH (and the Power)

4. Touch the left shoulder, and say/vibrate VE-GEDULAH (and the Glory)
5. Clasping both hands on the breast, say/vibrate LE OLAHM AMEN (forever, Amen)

Lesser Banishing Ritual of the Pentagram.

1. Face east. Stretch out right hand pointing with index finger and trace a banishing earth pentagram in visualized white light. "Stab it" in the center, and Vibrate YOD-HEH-VAV-HEH.
2. Turn south, with hand and finger still extended while visualizing a line of white light, then trace another pentagram of white light and stab it in the center, and vibrate AH-DOH-NAI.
3. Turn west, with hand and finger still extended and visualizing a line of white light, trace another pentagram of light and stab it, and vibrate EH-HEH-YEH.
4. Turn north and repeat drawing the circle and pentagram, stab it and vibrate AH-GE-LAH.
5. Return to face east, extend both arms to form a cross, and say: Before me Raphael, behind me Gabriel, on my right hand Michael, on my left hand Auriel, for before me flames the Pentagram, and behind me the Six-rayed Star.
6. Repeat the Kabbalistic Cross.

The ritual can be further developed by visualizing the Archangelic figures, in colored robes, at each station. Details can be found in the suggested readings.

The Middle Pillar. Standing, feet together, facing east:

1. Visualize a white sphere above the head and vibrate EH-HEH-YEH.
2. Visualize light descending to form a sphere at the throat, and vibrate YE-HOH-VOH E-LOH-HEEM.
3. Visualize light descending to form a sphere at the heart, and vibrate YE-HOH-VOH EL-OAH-VE-DA-ATH.
4. Visualize light descending to form a sphere at the genitals, and vibrate SHAH-DAI EL CHAI.
5. Visualize light descending to form a sphere at the feet, and vibrate AH-DOH-NAI HA-AH-RETZ.

6. Visualize and feel a current of light rising from the feet, entering the body at the base of the spine, and continuing upwards to flower out in a shower of light at the crown of the head, and then descend to re-enter at the feet. Continue to circulate the light at least four times.*

Repeat the Banishing Ritual and then close with the Kabbalistic Cross.

*Alternatively, and more traditionally, return attention to the center above the head and visualize a current descending from it to the left shoulder and then down inside the left side of the body to the sole of the left foot, and then over to the sole of the right foot and up through the right side of the body back above the head. Then do the same, only visualizing the current descending from the crown down the front of the body and then returning up from the feet and through the spine to the crown. Both currents should coincide with the breath, and should be repeated several times. A third circulation of the current is from beneath the right foot over to the left foot and then upward in a tight spiral about the entire body up to the center above the head.

Variations of the exercise with more details will be found in the suggested readings.

A similar approach involving six centers is practiced in the Aurum Solis system.

Suggesting reading: Regardie with the Ciceros: *The Middle Pillar: The Balance Between Mind and Magic*

—Regardie with the Ciceros: *A Garden of Pomegranates—Skrying on the Tree of Light*

—Regardie with the Ciceros: *The Tree of Life—An Illustrated Study in Magic*

—Denning and Phillips: *The Sword & The Serpent—The Two-Fold Qabalistic Universe*

Mind-Body Connection. (Self-Hypnosis) It is only recently that science has recognized that there is somewhat of a two-way street between Mind and Body. Both are far more complex than earlier perceived and more intimately connected through energy and hormonal exchanges. With this recognition, we have the beginning of 'mental healing' where visual images are found to influence the body. And, with meditation or hypnosis (and self-hypnosis, of course), imagined exercises and movements were found to result in muscular developments.

Suggested Reading: Reich, W.: *Character Analysis*

Equally interesting, with Reichian Therapy, deep massage and certain exercises involving specific muscle groups was found to release emotional traumas and bring memories of their origins to the conscious awareness.

Moon. (Tarot) The 18th Major Arcanum—image: a dog and a wolf by a body of water baying at the rising moon, or an owl flying beneath a full moon over water with swimming fish; Hebrew letter: Qoph; Divinatory meaning: delusion, the unknown, intuition; the 29th path on the Tree of Life .

Muladhara. (Etheric Body) The root chakra located at the base of spine, color red, associated planet Saturn, associated Sephirah: Malkuth.

Nephesh. (Kabbalah—Tree of Life) A part of the soul located in Yesod. The etheric body. It is the Lower Self or lower subconscious with primal instincts and drives.

Neshamah. (Kabbalah—Tree of Life) Located in Briah, it is one of the three highest parts of the soul along with Chiah in Chokmah and Yechidah in Kether that collectively compose the Higher Genius, the source of intuition.

Netzach. (Kabbalah—Tree of Life) The seventh Sephirah on the Tree of Life, Victory. It is located at the bottom of the Pillar of Mercy.
God Name: Tetragrammaton Tzaboath (Lord of Armies)
Archangels: Haniel (Grace of God)
Angelic Host: Tarshishim (Brilliant Ones)
Astrological Correspondence: Venus
Body: The left hip
Colors: in Atziluth: amber, in Briah: emerald, in Yetzirah: bright yellow green, in Assiah: olive flecked with gold
Consciousness: The Emotions, as part of Ruach (the Conscious Self)
Element: Fire
Magical Image: A beautiful naked woman
Symbol: The rose
Tarot: The four Sevens

New Age. A phrase adapted by certain occult writers to describe (1) A belief in a new level of consciousness coincident with the Aquarian Age. (2) A social movement of diverse spiritual and political elements directed toward the transformation of individuals and society through heightened spiritual awareness obtained through practices of meditation, yoga, ritual, and channeling. (3) A cultural phenomenon often associated with the psychedelic and mind-altering substances widely available in the 1960s.

It is an ideal of harmony and progress that includes feminist, ecological, holistic, and organic principles expressed through an alternative life style that developed its own music, fashions, communal living, open sexuality, and political activism.

It became a commercial category, particularly in the book trade, that brought together subjects related to self-understanding, self-transformation, and self-development including acupuncture, alchemy, ancient civilizations, angels, anthroposophy, aromatherapy, astral projection, astrology, Atlantis, auras, biofeedback, Buddhism, channeling, chanting, chakras, Chinese medicine, complementary healing, creative visualization, crystals, divination, dream interpretation, Egyptology, energy healing, ESP, extraterrestrial life, ghosts, Gnosticism, handwriting analysis, herbalism, hypnosis, Kabbalah, magick, martial arts, meditation, natural foods, numerology, occultism, organic gardening, Paganism, palmistry, paranormal phenomena, past lives, psychic healing, psychic powers, Reiki, reincarnation, runes, self-hypnosis, sex magick, shamanism, spiritual healing, Spiritualism, Tantra, Tarot, Theosophy, UFOs, Wicca, witchcraft, yoga, Zen, etc.

The New Age movement is inclusive of a resurgent paganism and rejection of formalistic religion in favor of Nature Mysticism and personal spirituality. While it generally includes roles for ministers and spiritual counselors along with those for priest and priestess as in Wicca, the religious aspect is participatory rather than hierarchical, ecstatic rather than puritanical, initiatory rather than theological, and inner-directed rather than outer. Divinity is found both within the person and in Nature, directly experienced rather than requiring an intermediary, and self-responsible rather than authoritarian.

While there are numerous organizations and groups, they are mostly informal, usually centered around lectures and workshops, and non-restrictive.

New Man. A belief, sometimes associated with the "New Age" (which see), that human evolution continues and is in the process of producing a new species with expanded awareness, various spiritual powers, more immunity to common diseases, longer lived, more altruistic, and consciousness-sharing. The New Man is less dependent upon governments, does not identify himself with race or nationality, is free of gender-bias, is mostly vegetarian, and is self-supportive.

New World Order. A 'World Order' is the overall structure of the intergovernmental networks of governance, the integration of national and regional economies, the role of international law, the play of communication, and the interrelationships of the dominant cultures. *When the existing order is dysfunctional, threatening to tear apart, a new order must replace the old.*

The current movement towards a new world order is seen by some as a continuation of the "new order for the ages" expressed in *Novus Ordo Seclorum,* which while forming part of the Great Seal of the United States is not limited historically or in concept to the United States. Thus, a 'new world order' or a 'new order for the ages' is perceived as evolutionary rather than limited to any previous or current governmental or economic system.

The New World Order must address the contemporary issues of religious conflict, a requirement for secular education, freedom from theocracy, dependence on natural resources, populism, a failing financial system and a failed monetary system, the need for international law and its enforcement outside of any nationalist base, an antiproductive and class-biased tax system, an antiquated health system, and many other derivative failures.

Novus Ordo Seclorum. The New Order of the Ages represented in the Great Seal of the United States. N.O.S. is the spiritual unity behind the nation and the container for all the ideas represented by its founding. It has the potential to function as the 'over soul' of the nation should people turn inward to its inspiration. As we turn to the N.O.S. for inner guidance it aligns the person with those high ideas and guides their translation into their practical and contemporary manifestation. It is the repository of the high aspirations of the Founding Fathers and those thinkers and leaders who have sought to create a *new* nation based on principles rather than geographic and tribal boundaries. It represents the Spirit of America.

Occult: That which is, at least temporarily, hidden from our perception. In astronomy it refers to the passing of one body in front of another as when the Moon passes in front of the Sun (an eclipse). In the common culture it has been used as a category for 'hidden' knowledge, i.e., those subjects and technologies functioning to manifest psychic and spiritual faculties.

Suggested Reading: Greer: *The New Encyclopedia of the Occult*

Operating System. (Self-Empowerment) Inside every computer there is a software package providing the instructions for the hardware to carry out the work requested by application software packages like Microsoft Word and Excel. The operating system is the interface between the computer hardware and the world, while the application packages are like the skills and training we learn by study and experience. Like every other computer the human brain requires an operating system that interfaces with the world and filters our perceptions to correspond to what we are conditioned to expect through parental guidance, our life experiences, education, training, and interaction with authority figures, social expectations, and to far lesser extent by our genetic heritage and past-life memories. This operating system also conditions and directs the way we respond to external stimuli. Much of this operating system functions in the subconscious mind. Like computers, the operating system can be modified, updated, changed, and even replaced. Self-understanding is learning about our operating system; self-improvement is about modifying and changing our operating system; self-transformation is about updating and largely replacing our operating system. The new science of Quantum Theory tells us that the beginning *is* (not just was *but still is*) the Universal Field of Possibilities that manifests first as Energy/Matter under the guidance of packets of information/instruction. Thus we can see an analogy with a computer with its Operating Program and its Application Programs.

Orgone. The universal life-force as conceived by Wilhelm Reich. Seemingly another name for odic force, prana, ether, mana.

Other-Directed Piscean Man. In contrast to the "Inner-directed Aquarian Man" (which see), the Other or Outer-directed person 'follows the crowd' and accepts the guidance of authority figures without reasonable questions. 'Inner-Directed' has also been associated with the Aquarian Age individual man in contrast to the Piscean Age with its symbolism of fish that swim in groups. The outer-directed person is perceived as easily manipulated because of his dependence on outer authority.

Paranormal. (Psychic Powers) Parallel to the normal. Phenomena that is beyond the understanding of material science. While the paranormal is mostly confined to psychic-type events and experience, it also includes certain physical phenomena for which we do not as yet have an explanation.

Past-Life Regression. (Self-Hypnosis) A technique involving hypnosis, self-hypnosis, or meditation to re-experience past-life events in order to resolve traumatic reactions, recover lost memories and skills, and resolve certain recurring problems.

Suggested Reading: Andrews: *How to Uncover Your Past Lives*

—Webster: *Practical Guide to Past Life Memories, Twelve Proven Methods*

Path-Working. (Kabbalah—Tree of Life) A guided visualization meditation between two Sephiroth on the Tree of Life.

Personal Responsibility. (Self-Empowerment) Acceptance of responsibility for personal acts and things controllable within one's personal life in contrast to dependence on Government and Society for personal welfare. It involves personal choices and decisions leading to greater independence rather than acceptance of perpetual dependence. "Seeking to improve oneself" is an example of personal choice. It is an essential decision for Self-Empowerment.

Personality. The immediate vehicle of personal consciousness we believe to be ourselves. It is a temporary complex drawn from the etheric, astral, and mental bodies containing the self-image, current life memories, and the current operating system. As the dictionary puts it: "*the totality of somebody's attitudes, interests, behavioral patterns, emotional responses, social roles, and other individual traits that endure over long periods of time.* (Encarta online dictionary copyright © 2008 Microsoft Corporation)

Physical Plane. The material plane of matter and energy as objective reality, and the end product of creation. But, even though it appears to us as solid, we have learned to understand it as space and energy, and we now know that it is subject to change under the direction of willed intention.

PK. (Psychic Powers) See Psychokinesis.

Planes. Different levels of existence and of consciousness. While there is debate on the total number and classification of the planes, the most common is that of the five planes as used in this book. From highest to lowest:
Spirit (sometimes considered as consisting of two additional
    planes)
Mind (commonly divided into Lower and Higher)
Astral (commonly divided into Lower and Higher)
Etheric (sometimes considered as two layers, one always attached
    to the physical and the other always to the astral)
Physical (sometimes with the lower part of the etheric attached)

Possession. The temporary displacement of the self by a spirit entity. Possession can be voluntary, as when a medium surrenders her/his body to a spirit, or involuntary when the entity takes over. In Voudoun, the god takes possession and 'rides' the person like a horse. While the person is possessed, the body is often capable of physical feats beyond the normal ability of the person.

A somewhat different situation arises when the control is involuntary. It becomes a state of possession in which a spirit or other entity, such as a "Loa" in the Voodoo religion. seems to push your conscious to one side and their consciousness takes over your body and personality.

Post-Hypnotic Cue. (Self-Hypnosis) A word, thought, image, or gesture presented during hypnosis, usually near the end of the trance, as a signal for later use to activate the full or certain specific empowering effects of the trance on demand. Synonym: post-hypnotic suggestion.

Post-Hypnotic Suggestion. (Self-Hypnosis) A suggestion given during hypnotic trance for action to be taken after the subject returns to normal consciousness, often intended to change one habit (a negative one) to another habit (a positive one).

Post-Script Cue. (Self-Hypnosis) A word, thought, image, or gesture presented during a script, typically near the end, for later use as a signal, typically to activate the full or certain specific empowering effects of the script on demand. Synonym: post-cue suggestion.

Power, The. Chi, Prana, Life Force, Kundalini. It refers in particular to the direction of personal energy combined with emotional force and conscious direct to bring about magical change.

Prana. Chi, the Force, the Power. The universal life energy flowing throughout the universe. It can be visualized as flowing into the body as you inhale, and then distributed throughout the body as you exhale.

Pre-Sleep Intervention. (Self-Hypnosis) The "Pre-sleep Intervention Program" is based on the premise that consciousness and subconsciousness, rather than simply categories or content areas, are complex mental processes that exist on a continuum that is receptive to our intervention.

Through pre-sleep intervention, you can tap into that continuum in ways that influence those processes. As a result, you access dormant potentials and activate them to achieve your personal goals. Beyond that, you can actually generate totally new potentials by taking command of the resources within. By perceiving consciousness and subconsciousness as a continuum, we are activating the 'whole person' rather than seeing division and separation. In the program, the most important step is before the beginning—that you really know what your goal is, or what your goals are. Only work with one at a time but know that it is a vitally important goal and truly <u>feel</u> its importance and value. Be willing to say to yourself that you are wholeheartedly <u>praying</u> for its realization.

Precognition. (Psychic Powers) The psychic awareness of the future, to include knowledge of events, trends, and conditions.

Premonition. (Psychic Powers) Like a 'hunch,' it is usually an advance warning, a presentiment of something undesirable that will occur in the future.

Psychic Attack. (Psychic Powers) An attack on the astral body that will cause an effect on the physical body as well. It may be intentional, but other times it is caused by strong emotions of hatred, greed, envy, lust, etc. directed towards the victim. See .

Psychic Body. (Etheric Body) Generally conceived as the Etheric and Astral bodies together.

Psychic Empowerment. (Psychic Powers) Generally the following of a specific plan or program, sometimes involving self-hypnosis and meditation, for the development of innate psychic powers into dependable skills. With empowerment, the psychic or spiritual bodies can be integrated into the whole person.

    Suggested Reading: Slate and Weschcke: *Psychic Empowerment for Everyone*

Psychic Powers. All the abilities, especially as trained skills, associated with the paranormal, including Astral Projection, Aura Reading, Channeling, Clairaudience, Clairvoyance, Extrasensory Perception, Mediumship, Mental Telepathy, Psychokinesis, Remote Viewing, Spirit Communication, Spiritual Healing, Telekinesis, Teleportation, etc.

    Suggested Reading: Denning and Phillips: *Practical Guide to Psychic Powers, Awaken Your Sixth Sense*

    —Webster: *Psychic Development for Beginners, An Easy Guide to Releasing and Developing Your Psychic Abilities*

    —Slate and Weschcke: *Psychic Empowerment for Everyone*

Psychic Self-Defense. (Psychic Powers) Techniques and practices to build psychic defenses against psychic predators, skilled advertisers and sales people, emotional manipulators, and psychic attack.

    Suggested Reading: Denning and Phillips: *Practical Guide to , Strengthen Your Aura*

    —Penczak: *The Witch's Shield, Protection Magick and*

Psychokinesis (PK). (Psychic Powers) The movement of objects without physical contact.

Psychometry. (Psychic Powers) The reading of emotional and psychic energies impressed on an object such as a watch, jewelry, etc. to reveal its history and ownership.

    Suggested Reading: Andrews: *How to Do Psychic Readings Through Touch*

Quantum Theory. The new science of Quantum Theory tells us that the beginning <u>is</u> (not just was *but still is)* the Universal Field of Possibilities that manifests first as Energy/Matter under the guidance of packets of information/instruction. Thus we can see an analogy with a computer with its Operating Program and its Application Programs.

Regression. (Self-Hypnosis) The recovery of past memories through hypnosis or meditation. To generate the regressed state, we use suggestions of traveling back in time to a stage of youthful prime. The program found that lingering in that regressed state of peak youthfulness tends to be rejuvenating.

Reincarnation. The belief that the Soul experiences multiple lives through newly born physical bodies and personalities. Upon death of the physical body, the personality withdraws to the astral and then mental plane while the essential lessons of that incarnation are abstracted to the Soul.

    Suggested Reading: Slate: *Beyond Reincarnation, Experience your Past Lives & Lives Between Lives*

    —Webster: *Practical Guide to Past Life Memories, Twelve Proven Methods*

    —Andrews: *How to Remember Past Lives*

Rejuvenation. (Self-Hypnosis) The condition of becoming youthful again, or the process of making a person young or youthful again. Aside from nutrition and sensible health care, the use of regression to an earlier time of peak youthfulness resets the aging clock.

    Suggested Reading: Slate: *Rejuvenation: Strategies for Living Younger, Longer & Better.* Book with audio CD

Repercussion. (Etheric Body) During astral, and more particularly, etheric projection, an injury to the projected subtle body can 'repercuss' back to injure the physical body. This includes not only possible psychic injury but damage done by certain metals including iron and silver. If a weapon of those metals is driven through the center of the projected body, i.e., the heart area, it can cause death. See Etheric Revenants (vampires) and Etheric Projection (werewolves).

Retrocognition. (Psychic Powers) Psychic knowledge of the past.

Rising on the Planes. (Kabbalah—Tree of Life) A Path-Working of rising up the Middle Pillar of the Tree of Life from Malkuth to Kether.

    Suggested reading: Regardie, with the Ciceros: *A Garden of Pomegranates—Scrying on the Tree of Life*

Rousing of the Citadels. (Meditation) An expanded version of the Middle Pillar Exercise involving the addition of a psychic center at the brow.

Suggesting reading: Denning and Phillips: *The Triumph of Light*

Ruach. (Kabbalah—Tree of Life) Breath, Spirit, the Conscious Self and middle part of the soul representing mind and reasoning power. It includes the five Sephiroth clustered at the central part of the Tree of Life: Chesed, Geburah, Netzach, and Hod, with Tiphareth at the center.

Runes. The ancient alphabet of the Germanic and Scandinavian peoples, used for both divinatory and magical purposes.

Suggested reading: Thorsson: *Northern Magic—Rune Mysteries and Shamanism*

—Aswynn: *Northern Mysteries & Magick—Runes & Feminine Powers*

Sahasrara. (Etheric Body) The chakra located at the crown above the head, color violet, associated planet none, associated Sephirah: Kether.

Scrying. An alternative spelling of Skrying, which see.

Séance. A group, usually as a circle, gathered together to give energy support to a person functioning as a 'medium' to serve as an intermediary in communication between the world of spirits of the deceased and living people.

Self. We distinguish between a little self (small 's') and a big Self (large 'S'). The small self is that of the personality, the person we think we are, and in fact are until we identify with the big Self that is also the 'Higher Self,' the permanent Self existing between incarnations.

Self-Confidence. (Self-Empowerment) Self-reliance. Belief in the ability of self to solve problems. Self-confidence is the catalytic force that empowers your newly developed inner resources to manifest in the outer world as Success.

Self-Development. (Self-Empowerment) The work, also called 'the Great Work,' of developing the little self into the big Self.

Self-Discovery. (Self-Empowerment) The discovery that there is a big Self that is different than the little self.

Self-Empowerment. A synthesis of Occultism, Psychology, and Self-improvement in a functional life style that is both practical and spiritual. Its goal is the fulfillment of the innate potentials leading to the whole person. Through the use of self-hypnosis, it condenses traditional esoteric programs by activating the subconscious mind and drawing upon the collective unconscious.

Self-Hypnosis. (Self-Hypnosis) The self-induction of hypnotic trance and the catalytic power of direct self-programming through simple but carefully developed affirmations mostly expressed as already accomplished "I AM" conditions, such as "I AM slim."

Suggested Reading: Park: *Get Out of Your Way, Unlocking the Power of Your Mind to Get What You Want.* Includes audio CD of self-hypnosis programs

Self-Improvement. (Self-Empowerment) We can always change for the better; we can improve ourselves physically, mentally, and spiritually; and no matter what the challenges may be, we can try to meet them on our own terms. Self-improvement starts with knowing where we are now and understanding how our current situation limits us. Then comes examination of where we can go from the current position and what steps we can make to move forward. And, finally, we see and accept the decisions to be made and the costs to be assumed.

Self-Knowledge. (Self-Empowerment) Self-knowledge means knowing just who you are—free of the gloss of what other people say and think, free of the bounds of family and place, and aware of the role of education and environment in your current conditioning.

Self-Programming. (Self-Empowerment) We make many programming choices, and the more understanding we have of the external programming placed upon us and knowing the opportunities we have to choose new programming, the greater our freedom to become more than we are.

Self-Talk, Self-Dialogue. (Self-Empowerment) Discussion with your self as if you are several people—which you are. Through such dialogue you isolate those different personae—masks—from one another until you know who you are and how you can make use of those different personae in your relationships with the outer world. You are the director and producer of the drama that is your life, and you are also all the main characters in the drama. They are the different personae that you can become at will as you gain knowledge and understanding.

Self-Understanding. (Self-Empowerment) Self-understanding is different from self-knowledge. Knowing who you are is different than understanding who you are. Understanding involves the "why" you are who you are—the karma leading up to now, the planetary factors in your horoscope, and the impact of your environment on who you are. Self-understanding also brings understanding of what the choices you have before you actually involve.

Sephirah. (Kabbalah—Tree of Life) Singular of Sephiroth. One of the ten divine states or emanations on the Tree of Life.

Sephiroth. (Kabbalah—Tree of Life) The ten sequential emanations of God that make up the divine states or energies on the Tree of Life. The names, meanings and astrological attributions are:

1. Kether	Crown	Primum Mobile
2. Chokmah	Wisdom	Zodiac, Sphere of the Stars
3. Binah	Understanding	Saturn
4. Chesed	Mercy	Jupiter
5. Geburah	Severity	Mars
6. Tiphareth	Beauty	Sun
7. Netzach	Victory	Venus
8. Hod	Glory	Mercury
9. Yesod	Foundation	Moon
10. Malkuth	Kingdom	Earth

Each Sephirah further contains an entire Tree of Life within itself, adding rich dimensions for meditation and exploration.

Seven Chakras. (Etheric Body) While there are many minor chakras, there are seven primary, as follows:

1. *Sahasrara,* crown, color violet, associated planet none, Sephirah: Kether.

2. *Ajna,* brow, color indigo, associated planet Moon, Sephiroth: Chokmah and Binah.

3. *Vishuddha,* throat, color blue, associated planet Mercury, Sephirah: Daath.

4. *Anahata,* heart, color green, associated planet Sun or Venus, Sephirah: Tiphareth.

5. *Manipura,* solar plexus below the navel, color yellow, associated planet: Mars, Sephirah: none suggested.

6. *Svadhisthna,* genital area, color orange, associated planet Jupiter or Moon, Sephirah: Yesod.

7. *Muladhara,* base of spine, color red, associated planet Saturn, Sephirah: Malkuth.

Seven Earths. (Kabbalah—Tree of Life) A Kabbalistic concept that there are seven earths, seven heavens, and seven hells. The seven earths are inhabited by humans or other intelligent beings. The names, experiences and corresponding Sephirah are:

1. Aretz	dry earth	the Supernals (Kether, Chokmah, Binah)
2. Adamah	red clay	Chesed
3. Gia	valley	Geburah
4. Neshiah	pasture	Tiphareth
5. Tziah	desert	Netzach
6. Arqa	seven hells	Hod
7. Thebel	earth and water	Yesod and Malkuth

Seven Heavens.

1. Araboth	plains	the Supernals (Kether, Chokmah, Binah)
2. Makhon	place	Chesed
3. Maon	residence	Geburah
4. Zebul	dwelling	Tiphareth
5. Shechaquim	clouds	Netzach
6. Raqia	firmament	Hod
7. Vilon	veil of heaven	Malkuth

Seven Hells.

1. Sheol	abyss	the Supernals (Kether, Chokmah, Binah)
2. Abbadon	destruction	Chesed
3. Bar Shachath	pit of ruin	Geburah
4. Tit ha-Yon	mire of mind	Tiphareth
5. Shaare Moth	gates of death	Netzach
6. Tzelmoth	shadow of death	Hod
7. Gehenna	valley of Hinnom	Yesod and Malkuth

Seven Rays. The primary creative energies of the universe and their technologies.

1. Red	Power	Shamanism
2. Blue	Wisdom	Meditation
3. Yellow	Intelligence	Astrology, Divination
4. Green	Beauty	Nature mysticism, Natural Living
5. Orange	Knowledge	Alchemy
6. Violet	Love	Devotional Mysticism
7. Indigo	Transcendence	Ceremonial Magic

Shadow. In Jung's psychology, the Shadow is a somewhat independent splinter personality representing those elements that have been deliberately or unconsciously repressed and denied expression in your life, or that are dormant and unrecognized. It is the Nephesh located in Yesod, the

Lower Self or lower subconscious with primal instincts and drives, most of which have been unconsciously banished in the drive for conformity and approval by the authorities in one's life.

With repressed elements there is a lot of emotional energy locked up. It's like prisoners in jail—human energy denied freedom. Sooner or later we need to confront these repressions and release those of childhood trauma, understand those repressed in the name of conformity, rationalize those that represent sensible behavior and customs, and get rid of the rest, while coming to terms with any that remain.

Yes, perhaps there is some inner 'demon' left that calls for professional help. Your subconscious will tell you if need be. Just listen for advice from your Inner Voice or Spirit Guide.

Shamanic Practices. The projection of conscious awareness into the astral world accomplished through trance induction by methods of physical stress including Fasting, Sleep Deprivation, Ecstatic Dancing, Flagellation, Prolonged Bondage, Sensory Deprivation, Sensory Overload, Drumming, and the use of hallucinogenic and psychoactive substances.

Suggesting Reading: Walsh: *The World of Shamanism, New Views of an Ancient Tradition*

Shape Shifting. (Etheric Body) The projection of the Etheric Body molded in the shape of an animal, or sometimes another person, to serve as a temporary vehicle for the lower self. See Etheric Projection and Etheric Revenants.

Shekinah. (Kabbalah—Tree of Life) In Kabbalah, the feminine aspect of God corresponding to Malkuth on the Tree of Life. Shekinah is the ever-continuing creative presence of God in the manifest universe.

Sigil. (1) The seal or abstract symbol evoking a spirit; (2) A personal ideogram condensing a written affirmation used to magically accomplish a particular objective. (3) A composition of English letters or geometric shapes symbolizing the magical goal upon which the magician concentrates during sexual orgasm to bring it into materialization.

Skrying. Sometimes spelled 'Scrying.' The psychic techniques of reaching into the subconscious mind by means of fascination devices such as crystal balls, magic mirrors, pendulums, etc., and focusing devices such as dowsing rods, shells, oracular dreaming, Ouija™ boards, aura reading, and psychometry, as an aid to concentration to allow visions and automatic writing and speaking, etc.

Suggested Reading: Tyson: *Scrying for Beginners, Tapping into the Supersensory Powers of Your Subconscious*

Skrying in the Spirit Vision. Skrying using a symbol. See Astral Doorways.

Sleeping Trance. (Self-Hypnosis) A Sleeping Trance is simply a trance state in which you have given over conscious control to another person, a god, spirit, guide, or 'control'—or a fragment of your own consciousness. You can put yourself into a sleeping trance as we will teach in this book: *Self-Empowerment through Self-Hypnosis.*

Soul. The essential self behind all personal manifestation. It is not the personality but it absorbs the core lessons learned in the life of each personality created in a series of incarnations.

Spark of Divinity. In our core of our consciousness, we have a spark of Divinity that gives us, in our Consciousness, the power to shape the future and even to change the present. We will earn that power through the techniques of Self-Empowerment and the Self-Improvement programs presented in this book.

Spirit. Used variously to identify (1) the Spiritual Body, or Soul; (2) the essence of the deceased person in communication with the living or appearing as a 'ghost;' (3) entities from other dimensions or planets channeling to humans; (4) nonhuman inhabitants of the astral plane; (5) a collective term for nonindividual spiritual power and intelligence, probably an aspect of the collective unconscious or universal consciousness; (6) the fifth element from which the lower four—Fire, Air, Water, and Earth—are derived. In addition, there is the 'Holy Spirit' that may be the Primal Consciousness or Matrix that can be activated by prayer or other affirmative thoughts.

Spirit Communication. Generally, the communication between living people and the spirits of the deceased. Also may include communication with other spiritual entities—Guides, Angels, Masters, etc.

 Suggested Reading: Buckland: *Buckland's Book of Spirit Communications*

 —Konstantinos: *Speak with the Dead, Seven Methods for Spirit Communication*

Spirit Guide. An entity manifesting on the astral or mental plane exhibiting high intelligence and wisdom with a personal interest in the welfare of the individual experiencing the more or less constant presence of the Guide.

 Suggested Reading—Andrews: *How to Meet and Work with Spirit Guides*

 —Webster: *Spirit Guides and Angel Guardians, Contact Your Invisible Helpers*

Spiritual Body. The highest aspect and consciousness of the human being.

Spiritual Plane. The highest level of creative being from which the lower planes are derived.

Spiritualism. Generally the practice and the religion associated with spirit mediumship and communication, and the belief in the survival of the individual after physical death as spirit.

Star. (Tarot) The 17th Major Arcanum—image: a bright star overhead and most commonly a naked woman kneeling at the edge of a body of water pouring water from two vessels, sometimes one onto the ground but other times both into the water; Hebrew letter: Tzaddi; Divinatory meaning: spiritual guidance, hope, help; the 28th path on the Tree of Life connecting Yesod to Netzach.

Strength. (Tarot) The 8th Major Arcanum—image: a woman allied with a lion; Hebrew letter: Teth; Divinatory meaning: the power to overcome obstacles; the 19th path on the Tree of Life connecting Geburah to Chesed.

Sub-Atomic Field. Also called simply 'the Field' in which primal/universal energy and matter appear as waves and then as particles when observed. It is the foundation for the study of Quantum Physics (also called Quantum Mechanics and Quantum Theory). Packets of energy/matter are called Quanta.

Subconsciousness. Also called 'the unconscious.' It is the *lower* part of the personality containing forgotten and repressed feelings and memories, and the fundamental belief or operating system that filters reality, that collection of guilt feelings called the 'Shadow,' the 'Anima' or 'Animus' collection of feelings representing our idealization or fear and hatred of the opposite gender, the various archetypes and mythic images formed through the history of human experience, all of which can operate as doorways or gates to the astral world and connect to the higher or super consciousness. The subconscious is also home to our instincts and the autonomic system that cares for the body and its operation. The subconscious mind is accessed by various techniques including hypnosis, prayer, and ritual, and during sleep.

Subconscious Mind. The subconsciousness—never asleep, always aware. The Nephesh.

Subconscious Resources. (Self-Empowerment) The subconscious, with communication to the collective unconscious and the super consciousness ,has very nearly unlimited resources available to you through your Guide.

Success Expectations. (Self-Empowerment) Success means 'goals accomplished.' Success is not only measured financially but by having met or exceeded your expectations and hopes in your endeavors. It can be found on the job, in your career, in your vocation, in your study program, in your hobby, in your relationships, and in your personal growth and development program. It is a strong and inclusive word. "I AM successful" is a dynamic and powerful affirmation. "You're a success" is a beautiful commendation. "Success Expectations" are what we create in connection with our goals, the carrot that pulls us forward. Always establish what your success expectations are and keep them in the forefront of your consciousness.

Sun. (Tarot) The 19th Major Arcanum—image: the Sun, usually with one or two children beneath in a walled garden and mostly including a horse; Hebrew letter: Resh; Divinatory meaning: success, healing, happiness; the 30th path on the Tree of Life connecting Yesod to Hod.

Super Conscious Mind. Your subconscious mind is mostly conditioned by the past, and your conscious mind by the present. But you were born with a basic purpose, with some specific learning goals for this lifetime. The super conscious mind is your doorway to and from the future. The super conscious mind is the higher self and the source of your inspiration, ideals, ethical behavior, and heroic action, and the very essence that is "the Light of Men" as it was in the beginning and as it is now and as it will always be . . . .

The super conscious mind is the *higher* level of personal consciousness with access to the universal of collective unconscious. It is where the 'gods' or powerful archetypes and spirit guides can be found, and where the Akashic Records are accessed.

Svadisthana. (Etheric Body) The sacral chakra located at the genital area, color orange, associated planet Jupiter or Moon, associated Sephirah: Yesod.

Symbols. (Meditation) It is through symbols and images, and icons, that we open the doors of our inner perception. The great secrets of magicians, shamans, and modern scientists are in the associations they attach to such icons, and in the power of certain signs and formulae to function as circuits and pathways—not in the brain but in consciousness.

Tantra. (Tantra) A very sophisticated and extensive system of ancient Indian Occultism from which many Eastern and Western practices are derived. Nevertheless, it has become most identified with (1) the Chakra system, (2) Kundalini, and (3) Sexual practices involving (a) extended intercourse, (b) complex positions and practices once considered 'deviant' such as anal intercourse, oral intercourse, and the consumption of an 'elixir' compounded of the masculine and feminine fluids sucked from the vagina after intercourse and shared by the two lovers, and {4} Worship of the partners, particularly the female, as the embodiment of Goddess and God.

Other occult principles and practices taken from Tantra include the Tattvas (the five basic elements and the twenty-five compounds visualized in meditation for psychic effects), Yantras (complex geometric diagrams of energy circuitry visualized in meditation for psychic effects), Mantras (chanting of sacred words and names in meditation for psychic effects), Yoga Nidra (visualizations of psychic energy movements within the body during meditation), and other esoteric practices.

Suggested Reading: Mumford: *A Chakra & Kundalini Workbook, Psycho-Spiritual Techniques for Health, Rejuvenation, Psychic Powers & Spiritual Realization*

—Mumford: *Yoga Nidra Meditation, Chakra Theory & Visualization.*—Audio CD with instruction booklet

Tarot. (Tarot) A vast system of Archetypal Knowledge condensed into a system of 78 images on cards that can be finger-manipulated and then laid out in systematic patterns to answer specific questions or provide guidance to the solution of problems. While it is a form of divination, it is one of the most sophisticated and carefully developed systems of images and relationships following the structure of the Kabbalah's Tree of Life. Going beyond divination, it is also a system to access the unconscious, and to structure magical ritual. It's a powerful Western esoteric system comparable to the Eastern I Ching.

Suggested Reading: Amber K and Azrael Arynn K: *Heart of Tarot, an Intuitive Approach*

—Ferguson: *The Llewellyn Tarot.* 78-card deck and 288-page book

—Ciceros: *The New Golden Dawn Ritual Tarot—Keys to the Rituals, Symbolism, Magic & Divination*

Tattwa (or Tattva). (Tantra) The five qualities or elements: Spirit, Fire, Air, Water, Earth. They are represented by five colored geometric diagrams used for meditation and as astral gateways. In addition, the five primary symbols are used to construct twenty-five compound symbols by placing a smaller image within a larger one to represent the general complexity of manifest life and form. The colors and shapes along with their Hindu names are:

Spirit	Akasha	Black	Oval egg
Air	Vayu	Blue	Circle
Fire	Tejas	Red	Triangle
Water	Apas	Silver	Crescent with horns upward
Earth	Prithivi	Yellow	Square

Telepathy. (Psychic Powers) See Mental Telepathy. Mind-to-mind communication or thought reading, more commonly experienced during trance.

Temperance. (Tarot) The 14th Major Arcanum—image: a woman pouring liquid from one vessel into another; Hebrew letter: Samech; Divinatory meaning: reconciliation, moderation; the 25th path on the Tree of Life connecting Yesod to Tiphareth.

Thought. Astral and mental combinations expressed mostly in words to represent a particular opinion, intention, or plan of action. We *think* thoughts. We *feel* emotions.

Thought Form. (Magick) (1) An astral image created by concentrated thought intended to accomplish a specified objective. When reinforced with emotion and charged with etheric energy, it will become physically manifest. (2) A spontaneous image created in the imagination that is charged with emotional energy. Either is perceived by a clairvoyant and is felt by ordinary people with some degree of psychic sensitivity. A carefully constructed mental image that is charged with emotional energy can become a manipulative tool used in product marketing, political action, and religious domination.

Suggested Reading: Ashcroft-Nowicki and Brennan: *Magical Use of Thought Forms, a Proven System of Mental & Spiritual Empowerment*

Three Levels of Consciousness.

I for Instinct, a function of the lower subconscious

I for Intelligence, a function of the ordinary consciousness

I for Intuition, a function of the super consciousness

Three Paths. (Kabbalah—Tree of Life) On the Tree of Life, three Paths lead upward from Malkuth—the Intellectual and Ceremonial path to Hod, the Emotional and Ritual Path to Netzach, and the Spiritual and Mystical Path to Yesod.

Three Pillars. (Kabbalah—Tree of Life) The three Pillars of the Tree of Life.

1. On the right, the Pillar of Mercy topped with Chokmah, then Chesed, and Netzach at the bottom. It is white, masculine, positive, and active—the Pillar of Force.

2. In the middle, the Pillar of Equilibrium, The Middle Pillar topped with Kether, then Daath, Tiphareth, Yesod, and Malkuth at the bottom. It is the Path of the Mystic, an Arrow straight from Malkuth to Kether, from the completion back to the Source. The Pillar of Mildness, of Balance.
3. On the left, the Pillar of Severity topped with Binah, then Geburah, and Hod at the bottom. It is black, feminine, negative, and passive—the Pillar of Form.

Three Principles. The three subtle substances that make up the basic composition of all matter. In Alchemy, they are referred to as Mercury, Salt, and Sulfur—but these are not the familiar substances of the same names but rather are like different states of all matter.

Tiphareth. (Kabbalah—Tree of Life) The sixth Sephirah on the Tree of Life, Beauty. It is located at the upper center of the Middle Pillar.
God Name: Tetragrammaton Eloah va-Daath (Lord God of Knowledge)
Archangel: Michael (He who is as God)
Angelic Host: Malakim (Kings)
Astrological Correspondence: Sun
Body: The solar plexus
Colors: in Atziluth: clear rose pink, in Briah: golden yellow, in Yetzirah: rich salmon pink, in Assiah: golden amber
Consciousness: The Imagination, as part of Ruach (the Conscious Self)
Element: Air
Magical Image: A naked child
Symbol: The truncated pyramid
Tarot: The four Sixes and the four Knights or Princes

Tower. (Tarot) The 16th Major Arcanum—image: struck by lightning with two persons falling from it; Hebrew letter: Peh; Divinatory meaning: danger, destruction, new beginning; the 27th Path on the Tree of Life connecting Hod to Netzach.

Training Programs. (Self-Empowerment) In Self-Empowerment it is necessary to train mind, memory, imagination, and visualization. Examples of simple programs to train the memory and the ability to visualize include:
Recreating your room. Simply look about the room you are in right now, and any time you have the opportunity in different rooms, then close your eyes and visually recreate it. With your eyes closed and looking at your imagined image of the room, pick our something significant

in all six parts of the room: ceiling, floor, and all four walls. Look for colors and shapes, note textures and the play of light and shadow. Estimate the room's measurements and the sizes of objects Play a game with yourself and pretend you are going to be paid money for everything accurately remembered.

Then open your eyes and look for those significant areas and see how well you did, and, even more importantly, how well you did with the areas adjacent to those significant areas. Repeat often. Later, when you are away from the room, close your eyes and recreate it again, and when you return, verify as many of the details as possible.

Self-Imaging. Take a simple statement, like "I AM slim," or "I AM strong," and picture yourself accordingly. Do not think of the process of becoming slimmer or stronger, but just a simple image that is you as stated. Now, write a description of what you saw, in detail. Repeat often.

Re-create an event. Think of a recent event at which you were present, and picture it in detail. See where you were and see what you were doing. See where other people were and what they were doing. Note what people are wearing, and especially jewelry and watches. Now, listen, and hear the sounds and voices of that event.

Re-create a story. Take a scene from a novel you recently read, and recreate the story in your imagination. Fill in the detail for what wasn't described in the printed version. Add sound effects, listen to the voices, and hear the sounds of the environment. Pretend that you are watching a movie made from the story and see the actors, see their hair, their clothes, how they move, feel their emotions.

Remember the day backwards. See yourself as you prepared to go to sleep, undressing from the day, having dinner, coming home from work, finishing up work, your work that day, etc., all the way back to having breakfast, dressing for the day, using the toilet, washing and showering, getting out of bed, and waking up. Note anything you wished you could change, and intentionally do so in your imagination. This especially concerns feelings where you have regret or even guilt for something said or done to others, and hurt and pain from things others said or did to you.

You don't *need* to carry pain or guilt around with you. Undo these matters in your imagination with strong feelings of intention to remove the pain, whether your or others. Such emotion is a barrier to your empowerment.

Create a Memory Palace. Don't use your own living quarters but create an apartment inside a building, and pretend you are both architect and interior designer. Construct and decorate a room for each major category of your life where you will store objects representing actual memories. Have a room representing marriage, for example, and start it with a wedding picture. Add memories using objects even if you have to imagine one, such as a photo you didn't take, and place it appropriately in the room.

Create another room representing your job, another for your hobby, another for each subject you've studied, and so on.

Now, keep adding memories to your palace. As you review your day, select things to be permanently 'filed' for future reference and create an 'icon' to contain everything important about each such thing.

Journal it. Nearly every self-improvement system, whether it is esoteric or mundane, recommends that you keep a journal or diary. Why? Because the act of recording 'solidifies' everything about the recorded event, and what you intend to do about it. If you regret something you said or did, record that you are un-doing it. If you are happy about something and want to affirm it, record that too.

Trance. (Self-Hypnosis) A state of consciousness in which awareness is concentrated, focused, and turned inward to the subconscious mind, either unconsciously through repetitive stimuli or consciously induced in a similar technique in hypnosis, meditation, or religious or shamanic practice. During a trance state, carefully constructed programs of suggestion and affirmation can lead to dramatic changes in conscious behavior and perceptions.

Tree of Life. (Kabbalah—Tree of Life) A diagram with ten spheres and twenty-two connecting paths that functions as a kind of 'Interdimensional' 'cross-indexing filing cabinet' for you to relate corresponding facts and experiences with others of the same nature along with the information similarly experienced and related by millions of other students over hundreds of years.

Triangle of Light. (Self-Hypnosis) The Triangle of Light is simply an equilateral triangle of light that you create in your imagination as you draw it with the index finger of your stronger hand. The physical act of drawing it gives 'substance' to the visualization.

Triangle of Power. (Self-Hypnosis) A physical gesture used to generate a triangle with the hands by joining the thumbs to form its base and the index fingers to form its peak. It is a multi-purposeful gesture that can be used to facilitate induction of self-hypnosis as well as to view the human aura, including that of oneself and others alike. It can also be used as a post-hypnotic or post-script cue.

Unconscious. (1) A lack of consciousness. (2) An alternate word for the subconscious mind. (3) A particular reference to the *personal* unconscious region of the mind where suppressed desires, memories, and feelings reside. In common usage, the personal unconscious is somewhat lesser than the subconscious mind. Some theoreticians believe that at least some psychic phenomena rise from these areas of the personality as *quanta* of energy/matter packets manifesting in poltergeist-like phenomena.

Universal Field of Possibilities. The Universal Field of Possibilities manifests first as Energy/Matter under the guidance of packets of information/instruction. Thus we can see an analogy with a computer with its Operating Program and its Application Programs. See Field.

Universal Force. The Force, the Tao, the Energy behind all existence, physical and otherwise.

Universe. (Tarot) The 21st Major Arcanum—image: a semi-naked woman surrounded by the Zodiac with animal images in the four corners representing the Elements; Hebrew letter: Tau; Divinatory meaning: the subject of the question and its place in the surrounding world; the 32nd path on the Tree of Life connecting Malkuth to Yesod.

Vibration. (Magick) When pronouncing a word or phrase for psychic effect, it must be done (1) at a lower octave than normal; (2) louder than normal but without stress; (3) with a vibratory feeling—sort of a trembling or buzzing sensation throughout the body. With practice the effect should be noticeable wherever the words are projected inside, or outside the body.

Vibratory Formula. (Self-Empowerment) Somewhat of an extension of the above but invoking divine energies and projecting them out to the universe.
1. Stand with arms extended to form a cross.
2. Draw in a deep breath.
3. Mentally pronounce the Divine Name as invoked from the heart.
4. Visualize the name descending to the energy center beneath the feet and then rising suddenly to the mouth.
5. Vibrate the name forcefully with the expulsion of the breath out the mouth.
6. See the Divine Name project to the furthermost reaches of the universe and then return to bathe the sender in its glory.

Visualization. (1) Creating a vivid image in your mind, before your closed eyes, or whatever is called for—a pictured object, person, word, symbol, alphabetical letter, deity, etc., making it glow, and then retaining that image as you open your eyes. (2) Using the imagination to create vivid images of desired conditions or objects to attract those goals. 'Creative Visualization' is a practical system for personal success.

Visualizing Scenes. The same process as above, but creating images of actual scenes rather than single objects. The scenes may be static or in motion depending upon the need.

Vishuddha. (Etheric Body) The chakra located at the throat, color blue, associated planet Mercury, associated Sephirah: Daath.

Vital Body. (Etheric Body) Same as the Etheric Body, which see.

Waking Trance. (Self-Hypnosis) Whenever you pay close attention to an idea, to conversation, to an object, and to your imagination, you are in an awake trance. The greater your depth of attention, the focus of your awareness, the deeper is your trance. The deeper is your trance, the more you are directing your consciousness to the object of your attention.

Wheel of Fortune. (Tarot) The 10th Major Arcanum—image: a wheel in the sky usually with eight directions marked out, and a variety of figures rising or falling on its rotation; Hebrew letter: Kaph; Divinatory meaning: transition, evolution, a change of fortune; the 21st path on the Tree of Life connecting Netzach to Chesed.

Whole Person. (Self-Empowerment) An expression to represent the entirety of our potential and inclusive of all the subtle bodies. In "becoming more than you are," you are fulfilling the innate potentials that you have. You are born a potentially whole and complete person, with undeveloped powers. The meaning of life is found in developing those powers, turning them into skills, and fulfilling all your potentials. That will make you a whole person.

Wholeness. (Self-Empowerment) The conscious mind and the subconscious mind, together, are the Lower Self while the super conscious mind is the Higher Self. Our goal is to link the two together in wholeness.

Will. Will is found in Geburah as part of Ruach, the Conscious Self. It is that part that decides on action and what that action will be, channeling all our energies towards a specific goal.

World. (Tarot) An alternate name for "Universe," the 21st Major Arcanum, which see.

Yantra. (Meditation) (Tantra) A particular geometric style of diagram from Tantric philosophy believed to represent and contain specific psychic energies. Meditation on the Yantra will induce specific consciousness experiences.

Yechidah. (Kabbalah—Tree of Life) The highest part of the soul, divine consciousness, located in Kether and part of the Neshamah, which see.

Yesod. (Kabbalah—Tree of Life) The ninth Sephirah on the Tree of Life, Foundation, located on the Middle Pillar between Tiphareth and Malkuth.

God Name: Shaddai El Chai (Almighty Living God)
Archangel: Gabriel (Strength of God)
Angelic Host: Kerubim (Powers of the Elements)
Astrological Correspondence: Moon
Body: The genitals
Colors: in : indigo, in Briah: violet, in Yetzirah: very dark
    purple, in Assiah: citrine flecked with azure
Consciousness: Thesubconscious mind, instincts, animal
    intelligence, the Nephesh
Element: Air
Magical Image: A handsome and strong naked man
Symbol: The truncated pyramid
Tarot: The four Nines

Yetzirah. (Kabbalah—Tree of Life) The third Kabbalistic world. The astral and angelic world of formation. The etheric matrix behind the material universe. Yetzirah corresponds to the seventh through ninth sephiroth: Netzach, Hod, and Yesod.

APPENDIX A

SELF-EMPOWERMENT JOURNAL
AND MAGICAL DIARY

(Your Name) _____

Date: _____ Day of Week: _____

Moon Phase: _____ Moon Sign: _____

Year—Month—Date_____ 1st, 2nd, 3rd, 4th

Schedule—Significant Events to think about: _____

_____

_____

Day's Events, *Remembering backwards*—We've broken the day into |
    twelve logical segments to aid the process.

Night: _____

_____

After Dinner: _____

_____

Dinner: _____

_____

After Work: _____

_____

Work: _____

_____

Lunch: _____

Work: _____

_____

Before Work: _____

_____

Breakfast: _____

_____

Before Breakfast: _____

_____

Getting Up: _____

_____

Diary—Significant Events: _____

_____

Dream—Description: _____

_____

_____

_____

Analysis: _____

_____

_____

_____

Significant Symbols: _____

_____

_____

_____

Meaning: _____

_____

_____

_____

_____

_____

_____

Health—Significant Factors: _____

_____

Healing Insights: _____

_____

Intentions: _____

_____

Prayers, Rituals, or Adorations: _____

_____

Self-Empowerment Exercises—Program Name: _____

_____

Event: _____

_____

Time Started: _____

Time Finished: _____

Results: _____

_____

_____

_____

_____

_____

Meaning: _____

_____

_____

_____

_____

Meditations: _____

_____

_____

_____

_____

_____

Insights: _____

_____

_____

_____

Interventions and Paranormal Events: _____

_____

Insights: _____

_____

_____

_____

Books read: _____

_____

Insights: _____

_____

_____

_____

Important Conversations: _____

_____

Self-Discoveries: _____

_____

_____

_____

Planning Ahead: _____

_____

_____

_____

_____

_____

Appendix B

THE KEY STEPS IN THE INDUCTION PROCESS

Preparation

Identify. Before selecting a problem or goal for your Self-Hypnosis intervention, it is important that you identify what it is that you really want. Go into your general meditation procedure and ask to see yourself as you want to be. Don't be in a hurry, and don't presume that you already know the important problems or goals. Ask questions and let your subconscious give you some answers. If there are not immediate responses, ask yourself questions about the self-image you want to see in relation to health, appearance, career, relationships, family, etc. Find two or three important self-images expressing particular problems or goals, and decide which the most important one is now, and keep the rest for later.

The Problem. Knowing what you really want, select a problem to resolve or a goal for action, such as losing weight. Make your goal reasonable. If it is too grand, you may lose confidence in its attainment. There should be no doubt in your mind that it can be done. If necessary, break a larger goal down into a series of logical shorter goals, but be careful not to minimize the process.

It is better to focus on a single goal at a time, or you can add two or three closely related subgoals to it. Make sure that the subgoals support the major goal.

Write it down. Write down your reasons for taking action. Build a solid case, and show the benefits. Following our example of weight loss, it might be for health reasons or for appearance. Be specific and justify the program. For most people, a present weight of 300 pounds is hard on the heart, on the knees, on the pancreas, etc. It may also be difficult to find attractive clothing. That much weight is probably fatiguing. So much weight may affect your sleep, even causing sleep apnea. And if your doctor or your spouse is telling you to lose weight, write that down as well. Convince yourself of the desirability of your goal.

Analyze the Challenge. You have a problem, and you know the reasons to make the change. But, if that was all there was to it, you would have solved the problem long ago. You have to ask yourself why it is that you still have the problem, in this example, overweight. Deep inside, in your subconscious, there are reasons you overeat despite your desire to be physically fit and attractive. Why do you do something that *rationally* you know that you should not?

Be honest in digging up those answers; some of them may be embarrassing; some of them may be hurtful—but it's important to understand the origins of the problem in order to change from old to new. The reasons for change outweigh the old reasons that caused the problem, but you have to see them for what they are—old, tired illusions.

Write them down right next to the reasons to change, and see how the new cancel out the old.

Write your expectations. Write down your expectations for results. Look into the future and see yourself as you want to be, and see all that it involves. In regard to the example weight problem, are there particular factors that you need to acknowledge as difficulties to be overcome?

Write the I AM sentence. Write a short, single sentence starting with "I AM" that expresses the successful outcome of the Self-Hypnosis you are about to undertake. An example would be: "I AM slim." Always keep the "I AM" in capital letters. This is a statement of the goal accomplished, of the new reality that has replaced the old.

Memorize it. Say it to yourself in a way that *feels* meaningful and powerful. Speak the words out loud and listen to them, and memorize the sound, the inflection, and the feeling. Then say it silently while hearing it in your head with the same feelings as when spoken out loud. Say it with energy. Say it with certainty that it already is. You will say it silently with your inner voice.

Visualize it. Close your eyes and visualize the sentence in White Letters against a black background. As you see it, speak the sentence with your inner voice.

See it now. Build a picture of the future in which your problem is resolved, your goal attained. Remember: You are leaving the old reality behind and see yourself already living in the new reality. See it, feel it, think it, believe it—you are there now. You are in the new reality. Write it down.

APPENDIX C

MEDITATION GUIDELINE

Comfort and Security. Make yourself comfortable and arrange things so you will not be disturbed except for a genuine emergency. Sit either upright or partially reclining, but do not lie down unless that's a physical necessity for you. Dim the lights to a comfortable level. It is preferable that you do not have incense burning or background music or a soundtrack, except as will be discussed later. You want to avoid the distraction that these otherwise niceties can provide.

Relaxation. Do your regular relaxation to enter into meditation. One very powerful procedure is called "Tension and Release," made up of the following steps:

Tense all muscles. Take a deep breath and hold it while tensing all your muscles, from head to toe, including the facial muscles. Feel the muscle contraction in your jaw, around your eyes, even around your ears, feel it in your neck and shoulders, chest and arms, make fists, feel the contraction in your chest, abdomen, groin, upper thighs, knees, and calves, and point your toes. Hold your body with all the muscles in deep tensions until you have to let your breath out, and then relax as you breathe out completely, letting go of all tension, mind chatter, and emotional concerns.

An alternative is called 'fractional relaxation' where you tense first your toes and then release, then your foot and release, progressing up the body all the way to the scalp. After you've done it a few times, you will be amazed at how fast and how completely you will relax the whole body.

Breathe fully and regularly. Breathe deeply, in and out, in and out, again and again. Feel and see the oxygen-rich air filled with life energy filling your lungs and spreading throughout your body. Then as you exhale, feel and see the out-breath carrying away waste products. Your body feels refreshed, healed, and deeply relaxed. Feel yourself fully cleansed physically and mentally.

Finding the center. Continue the regular breathing, continue feeling cleansed and relaxed, and a moment will come when you feel yourself experiencing an inner awakening, opening like a flower into full receptivity. Continue enjoying this blissful state, feeling calmness, vitality, peacefulness, and strength, ready to receive your self-instruction.

See and Hear your I AM sentence. When ready, see your memorized sentence in white letters against a black background in your Mind's Eye. Hold that vision for about two minutes (Do not count seconds and do not open your eyes to check the actual time. Just do it until you feel satisfied) while silently saying the sentence slowly with feeling and inflection. Listen to your inner voice and hear it with your inner ears so it seems just as if you were hearing it aloud.

Image or Symbol. Now, silently ask your subconscious mind to produce a simple image or symbol to fully represent that sentence. If nothing comes to you, repeat daily until it does. (There is a difference between an image and a symbol. A symbol is usually something already existing, often a three-dimensional object, with particular ideas and energies associated with it. Those ideas and energies must be in harmony with your I AM sentence to work effectively for you. An image is usually a simple picture or visual pattern created by your subconscious to work with your "I AM" sentence.) Memorize it, and draw it—no matter what your artistic skills are.

Memorize it. See your Image or Symbol in the same mental scene as your "I AM" sentence. Know that you now have the power to make your dream come true, the power to realize your goal, the power to make it your new reality replacing the old reality.

The New Reality. Remember that we are not merely leaving old habits behind but an old reality and replacing it with a new reality that is your own. Think about yourself in the future that will be after you have solved your problem, after you have fulfilled your goal. See yourself in this new reality as if it has already happened. Make this your future NOW. Feel yourself in the new reality, repeat your vision of the image and your "I AM" sentence together, and hear your inner voice say it. Tie it all together so any time you repeat the sentence in your mind you know that what is accomplished in the Inner World is manifesting in the physical world, and that your Body, Mind, and Spirit are working together to bring this about.

Appendix D

EXAMPLE SCRIPT OUTLINE

Step 1. Goal Statement. Formulate your goal of developing your mediumistic potentials and using them to empower your life.

Step 2. Focused Attention and Receptivity. Induce a state of focused attention and receptivity to suggestion, either through self-hypnosis or some other referred option, such as meditation, deep relaxation, or the drowsy state preceding sleep.

Step 3. Self-Empowerment Dialogue. While in the deeply focused and receptive state, initiate positive self-dialogue related to the development and application of your mediumistic potentials.

Step 4. Visualization.

Step 5. Affirmation. Affirm your strong commitment to use your new skills.

Step 6. Post-script Cue. Give yourself the post-script cue that you can at any moment activate your skills by visualizing a symbol, gesture, or other cue.

Step 7. Exit and Conclusion. Conclude this script by giving yourself permission to exit the trance or other receptive state. Take time to reflect on the information gained during the experience and your sense of spiritual empowerment. Record your experience.

Index